OXFORD ASSESS AND PROGRESS
EMERGENCY MEDICINE

Pawan Gupta

Consultant, Clinical Director, and Clinical Teacher
East & North Hertfordshire University Trust
Lister Hospital, Stevenage and
Queen Elizabeth II Hospital,
Welwyn Garden City

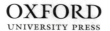

OXFORD
UNIVERSITY PRESS

OXFORD
UNIVERSITY PRESS

Great Clarendon Street, Oxford OX2 6DP

Oxford University Press is a department of the University of Oxford.
It furthers the University's objective of excellence in research, scholarship, and
education by publishing worldwide in

Oxford New York

Auckland Cape Town Dar es Salaam Hong Kong Karachi
Kuala Lumpur Madrid Melbourne Mexico City Nairobi
New Delhi Shanghai Taipei Toronto

With offices in

Argentina Austria Brazil Chile Czech Republic France Greece
Guatemala Hungary Italy Japan Poland Portugal Singapore
South Korea Switzerland Thailand Turkey Ukraine Vietnam

Oxford is a registered trade mark of Oxford University Press
in the UK and in certain other countries

Published in the United States
by Oxford University Press Inc., New York

© Oxford University Press, 2011
Reprinted 2014, 2016, 2019

British Library Cataloguing in Publication Data

Data available

Library of Congress Cataloguing in Publication Data

Data available

Typeset in ITC Charter
by Glyph International, Bangalore, India
Printed in China by
C&C Offset Printing Co. Ltd.

ISBN 978–0–19–959953–0

10 9 8 7 6 5 4

SERIES EDITOR PREFACE

The Oxford Assess & Progress Series is a groundbreaking development in the extensive area of self-assessment texts available for medical students. The questions were specifically commissioned for the series, written by practising clinicians, extensively peer reviewed by students and their teachers, and quality assured to ensure that the material is up to date, accurate, and in line with modern testing formats.

The series has a number of unique features and is designed as much as a formative learning resource as a self-assessment one. The questions are constructed to test the same clinical problem-solving skills that we use as practising clinicians, rather than just testing theoretical knowledge, namely:

- Gathering and using data required for clinical judgement
- Choosing examination, investigations, and interpretation of the findings
- Applying knowledge
- Demonstrating diagnostic skills
- Ability to evaluate undifferentiated material
- Ability to prioritize
- Making decisions and demonstrating a structured approach to decision making.

Each question is bedded in reality and is typically presented as a clinical scenario, the content of which have been chosen to reflect the common and important conditions that most doctors are likely to encounter both during their training and in exams! The aim of the series is to build the reader's confidence around recognizing important symptoms and signs and suggesting the most appropriate investigations and management, and in so doing aid development of a clear approach to patient management which can be transferred to the wards.

The content of the series has deliberately been pinned to the relevant Oxford Handbook but in addition has been guided by a blueprint which reflects the themes identified in *Tomorrow's Doctors* and *Good Medical Practice* to include novel areas such as history taking, recognition of signs including red flags, and professionalism.

Particular attention has been paid to giving learning points and constructive feedback on each question, using clear fact or evidence-based explanations as to why the correct response is right and why the incorrect responses are less appropriate. The question editorials are clearly referenced to the relevant sections of the accompanying Oxford Handbook and/or more widely to medical literature or guidelines. They are designed to guide and motivate the reader, being multi-purpose in nature, covering, for example, exam technique, approaches to difficult subjects, and links between subjects.

Another unique aspect of the series is the element of competency progression from being a relatively inexperienced student to a more experienced junior doctor. We have suggested the following four degrees of difficulty to reflect the level of training so the reader can monitor their own progress over time, namely:

★   Graduate should know

★ ★   Graduate nice to know

★ ★ ★   Foundation should know

★ ★ ★ ★   Foundation nice to know.

We advise the reader to attempt the questions in blocks as a way of testing knowledge in a clinical context. The series can be treated as a dress rehearsal for life on the ward by using the material to hone clinical acumen and build confidence by encouraging a clear, consistent, and rational approach, proficiency in recognizing and evaluating symptoms and signs, making a rational differential diagnosis, and suggesting appropriate investigations and management.

Adopting such an approach can aid not only being successful in examinations, which really are designed to confirm learning, but more importantly being a good doctor. In this way we can deliver high-quality and safe patient care by recognizing, understanding, and treating common problems, but at the same time remaining alert to the possibility of less likely but potentially catastrophic conditions.

David Sales and Kathy Boursicot, Series Editors
November 2010

A NOTE ON SINGLE BEST ANSWER AND EXTENDED MATCHING QUESTIONS

Single best answer questions are currently the format of choice being widely used by most undergraduate and postgraduate knowledge tests, and hence most of the assessment questions on this book follow this format.

Briefly, the single best answer question presents a problem, usually a clinical scenario, before presenting the question itself and a list of five options. Of these five, there is one correct answer and four incorrect options or 'distracters' from which the reader chooses a response.

Extended matching questions are also known as extended matching items and were introduced as a more reliable way of testing knowledge. They are still currently widely used in many undergraduate and postgraduate knowledge tests, and hence are included in this book.

An extended matching question is organized as one list of possible options followed by a set of items, usually clinical scenarios. The correct response to each item must be chosen from the list of options.

All of the questions in this book, which typically are based on an evaluation of symptoms, signs, or results of investigations either as single entities or in combination, are designed to test *reasoning* skills rather than straightforward recall of facts, and use cognitive processes similar to those used in clinical practice.

The peer-reviewed questions are written and edited in accordance with contemporary best assessment practice and their content has been guided by a blueprint pinned to all areas of *Good Medical Practice*, which ensures comprehensive coverage.

The answers and their rationales are evidence based and have been reviewed to ensure that they are absolutely correct.

Incorrect options are selected as being plausible and indeed may look correct to the less knowledgeable reader. When answering questions, readers may wish to use the 'cover' test in which they read the scenario and the question but cover the options.

Kathy Boursicot and David Sales, Series Editors

PREFACE

'To study the phenomenon of disease without books is to sail an uncharted sea, while to study books without patients is not to go to sea at all.'

Sir William Osler, Professor of Medicine, Oxford

Assessment in medicine has, in the course of time, evolved from simple, descriptive essay-type questions through multiple true/false to a more specific application of knowledge by way of single best answer (SBA) and extending matching questions (EMQ) in the setting of clinical situations.

This book is unique as it includes questions and answers on various aspects of emergency medicine, a specialty that has seen a rapid and vigorous expansion and recognition internationally in recent times. Today, emergency medicine covers a bewilderingly wide spectrum of problems ranging from the common ones seen in day-to-day practice to rare but potentially life-threatening diseases which can even catch experienced clinicians by surprise (but should not to be missed by any means). The identification as well as stabilization of a life- or limb-threatening condition in a patient within a time-constrained situation requires a systematic approach by emergency medicine clinicians.

This book, through the framework of SBAs and EMQs, provides examples of the most systematic approach to such emergencies. The questions presented in this book are primarily referenced to the *Oxford Handbook of Emergency Medicine* and its chapter layout closely follows the same. The answer to each question is followed by a rationale for the correct choice and an explanation as to why the other options are incorrect/inappropriate. Every effort has been rendered to provide an evidence-based bio-scientific explanation derived from the latest high-quality literature. The book has been carefully and sufficiently enriched with the latest external references and relevant national guidelines. An expansive literature on emergency medicine, such as the Oxford Handbook series, *Rosen's Emergency Medicine*, etc. have been thoroughly ransacked for condensing the enormous mass of information to the very essentials. The questions are based on clinical scenarios, most of them taken from real-life experiences and lessons learnt from near-misses made by various grades of doctors and nurse-practitioners while assessing and treating patients in the emergency department. The questions also cover the practical skills that are widely employed across emergency departments in the UK, and the issues related to medical ethics, training, and teaching, as well as the basics of disaster management. Photographs (provided in colour at the book's Online Resource Centre), and several X-rays and ECGs have been provided where relevant to highlight certain complex situations in clinical context.

The aim of this book is not to facilitate cramming of the questions by readers just for a successful result in the final examinations, but to provide a platform for starting on a stimulating, enjoyable, and thought-provoking experience, so that this book may be used by the reader as a reference even in future clinical practice.

Pawan Gupta

ACKNOWLEDGEMENTS

I would like to thank Dr David Sales, not only as a series editor, but also for placing his trust in my abilities and giving me the opportunity to help young doctors or would-be doctors in preparation for their future. I am grateful to Caroline Connelly, Philippa Hendry, Holly Edmundson, and Geraldine Jeffers for their support and guidance. I am indebted to the authors of the *Oxford Handbook of Emergency Medicine* for enabling this work to be linked to their book and to be referenced for providing feedback to the readers. I would like to thank the staff of the library at Lister Hospital, Stevenage, Hertfordshire, for their help in providing me with relevant literature and books for this project.

I am also grateful to the following colleagues who gave me invaluable advice for material included in some chapters: Mr Rajesh Varma, Consultant Obstetrician and Gynaecologist, Guy's and St. Thomas' NHS Foundation Trust, London; Dr Oyedeji Ayonrinde, Consultant Psychiatrist and Honorary Clinical Senior Lecturer, South London and Maudsley NHS Foundation Trust, London; Dr Donald C Brown, Honorary Senior Lecturer in Paediatrics, University of Edinburgh; and Mrs Mary Emson, Named Child Protection Nurse, East & North Hertfordshire NHS Trust, Stevenage.

My thanks also to the external reviewers, both medical students and specialists whose comments and challenges have helped me in improving my original ideas.

Finally, I am grateful to my entire family for their constant support, encouragement, and patience in making this effort a success.

FIGURE
ACKNOWLEDGEMENTS

I am grateful to all the patients and their relatives who have given me permission to publish their images to be used in this book. I am also thankful for the following permissions:

Figure 3.9: http://pediatriceducation.org © 2003–2010 Donna M. D'Alessandro, M.D. and Michael P. D'Alessandro, M.D.; **Figure 3.26**: Nunn AJ, Gregg I (1989) New regression equations for predicting peak expiratory flow in adults, *BMJ* **298**;1068–70; **Figure 3.27**: MacDuff A, Arnold A, Harvey J, *et al.* (2010) Management of spontaneous pneumothorax: British Thoracic Society pleural disease guideline 2010, *Thorax* **65** (Suppl 2):ii18eii31, © British Thoracic Society; **Figure 4.2**: © Dr Alun Hutchings, Cardiff Toxicology Laboratories; **Figure 7.1**: Copyright © MyFootShop.com™; **Figures 11.1, 11.3, and 11.5**: © 1998–2010 Ted M. Montgomery; **Figure 11.2** © 1994–2010 WebMD LLC; **Figure 11.4** © Dr Thomas Margius, http://www.eyedoctom.com; **Figure 14.1**: Hassan TB, *et al.* (1999) Algorithm for the management of a patient admitted with self poisoning or deliberated self harm who refuses treatment and is at risk of harm *BMJ* **319**: 107–9; **Figures 15.3 and 15.4**: Milner RDG and Herber SM (1990) *Diagnostic Picture Tests in Paediatrics*, Wolfe Publishing Ltd; **Figures 15.11 and 15.12**: Advanced Paediatric Life Support Manual (Advanced Life Support Group) **Appendix 1**: © Resuscitation Council (UK) 2008; **Appendices 2–8**: © Resuscitation Council (UK) 2010; **Appendix 9**: Teasdale G, Jennett B (1974) Assessment of coma and impaired consciousness: A practical scale, **Lancet 2**:81–84.

Reproduced with permission from Oxford University Press: **Figure 3.25**: Myerson *et al.*, *Emergencies in Cardiology*, 2nd edn, page 43, Figure 6.1; **Figure 3.28**: Wyatt, *Oxford Handbook of Emergency Medicine*, 3rd edn, figure on the inside backcover; **Figures 3.29 a and b**: Longmore *et al.*, *Oxford Handbook of Clinical Medicine*, 8th edn, pages 452 and 453; **Figure 3.30**: Longmore *et al.*, *Oxford Handbook of Clinical*

Medicine, 8th edn, page 813; **Figure 8.4**: Wyatt, *Oxford Handbook of Emergency Medicine*, 3rd edn, page 389; **Figure 9.13**: Wyatt, *Oxford Handbook of Emergency Medicine*, 3rd edn, pages 384 and 385; **Figure 12.1** Collier *et al.*, *Oxford Handbook of Clinical Specialties*, 8th edn, page 575; **Figure 15.9**: Wyatt, *Oxford Handbook of Emergency Medicine*, 3rd edn, page 637; **Figure 15.10**: Wyatt, *Oxford Handbook of Emergency Medicine*, 3rd edn, page 641; **Figure 15.13**: Wyatt, *Oxford Handbook of Emergency Medicine*, 3rd edn, page 715; **Figure 15.14**: Collier *et al.*, *Oxford Handbook of Clinical Specialties*, 8th edn, page 107; **Figure 15.15**: Wyatt, *Oxford Handbook of Emergency Medicine*, 3rd edn, page 674.

CONTENTS

NORMAL AND AVERAGE VALUES

	Normal value
Haematology	
White cell count (WCC)	$4-11 \times 10^9/L$
Haemoglobin (Hb)	M: 13.5–18g/dL F: 11.5–16g/dL
Packed cell volume (PCV)	M: 0.4–0.54% F: 0.37–0.47%
Mean corpuscular volume (MCV)	76–96fL
Neutrophils	$2-7.5 \times 10^9/L$
Lymphocytes	$1.3-3.5 \times 10^9/L$
Eosinophils	$0.04-0.44 \times 10^9/L$
Basophils	$0-0.1 \times 10^9/L$
Monocytes	$0.2-0.8 \times 10^9/L$
Platelets	$150-400 \times 10^9/L$
Reticulocytes	$25-100 \times 10^9/L$
Erythrocyte sedimentation rate (ESR)	<20mm/h (but age dependent; see OHCM p356)
Prothrombin time (PT)	10–14s
Activated partial thromboplastin time (aPTT)	35–45s
International normalized ratio (INR)	0.9–1.2
Biochemistry	
Alanine aminotransferase (ALT)	5–35IU/L
Albumin	35–50g/L
Alkaline phosphatase (ALP)	30–150U/L
Amylase	0–180U/dL
Aspartate transaminase (AST)	5–35IU/L
Bilirubin	$3-17\mu mol/L$
Calcium (total)	2.12–2.65mmol/L

Chloride	95–105mmol/L
Cortisol	450–750nmol/L (am) 80–280nmol/L (midnight)
C-reactive protein (CRP)	<10mg/L
Creatine kinase	M: 25–195IU/L F: 25–170IU/L
Creatinine	70-<150µmol/L
Ferritin	12–200µg/L
Folate	2.1µg/L
γ-Glutamyl transpeptidase (GGT)	M: 11–51IU/L F: 7–33IU/L
Lactate dehydrogenase (LDH)	70–250IU/L
Magnesium	0.75–1.05mmol/L
Osmolality	278–305mOsmol/kg
Potassium	3.5–5mmol/L
Protein (total)	60–80g/L
Sodium	135–145mmol/L
Thyroid stimulating hormone (TSH)	0.5–5.7mu/L
Thyroxine (T$_4$)	70–140nmol/L
Thyroxine (free)	9–22pmol/L
Urate	M: 210–480µmol/L F: 150–39µmol/L
Urea	2.5–6.7mmol/L
Vitamin B$_{12}$	0.13–0.68mmol/L
Arterial blood gases	
pH	7.35–7.45
PaO$_2$	>10.6kPa, 75–100mmHg
PaCO$_2$	4.7–6.0kPa, 35–45mmHg
Bicarbonate	24–28mmol/L
Base excess	±2mmol/L
Urine	
Cortisol (free)	<280nmol/24h
Osmolality	350–1000mOsmol/kg
Potassium	14–120mmol/24h
Protein	<150mg/24h
Sodium	100–250mmol/24h

ABBREVIATIONS

AAA	abdominal aortic aneurysm
ABC(DE)	airway, breathing, circulation, (disability, exposure)
ACS	acute coronary syndrome
ACTH	adrenocorticotropic hormone
AF	atrial fibrillation
AIDS	acquired immunodeficiency syndrome
AIS	abbreviated injury scale
ALP	alkaline phosphatase
ALT	alanine aminotransferase
AP	anteroposterior
APTT	activated partial thromboplastin time
ASA	American Society of Anesthesiologists
AST	aspartate aminotransferase
ATLS	advanced trauma life support
AV	atrioventricular
AV(N)RT	atrioventricular nodal re-entrant tachycardia
BE	base excess
BNF	*British National Formulary*
BP	blood pressure
bpm	beats per minute
C	Celsius
CABG	coronary artery bypass graft
CAMHS	children and adolescent mental health service
CCU	coronary care unit
CK-MB	creatinine kinase MB isoenzymes
cm	centimetre
CMV	cytomegalovirus
CO	carbon monoxide
CO_2	carbon dioxide
COPD	chronic obstructive pulmonary disease
CPAP	continuous positive airway pressure
CPR	cardiopulmonary resuscitation
Cr	creatinine

CRP	C-reactive protein
CSF	cerebrospinal fluid
CT	computed tomography
CVS	cardiovascular system
DC	direct current
DCS	decompression sickness
DKA	diabetic ketoacidosis
DPL	diagnostic peritoneal lavage
ECG	electrocardiogram
ED	emergency department
EMQ	extended matching question
ENT	ear, nose, and throat
ESR	erythrocyte sedimentation rate
FAST	focused assessment with sonography for trauma
FiO_2	inspired oxygen concentration
fL	femtolitre
FY1/2	foundation year 1/2
g	gram
G	gauge
GA	general anaesthesia
GABA	γ-aminobutyric acid
GBS	group B streptococcus
GCS	Glasgow Coma Scale
GI	gastrointestinal
GP	general practitioner
GTN	glyceryltrinitrate
$H_{1/2}$	histamine type 1/2
h	hour
HCG	human chorionic gonadotropin
HCO_3	bicarbonate
Hg	mercury
Hib	*Haemophilus influenzae* type b
HIV	human immunodeficiency virus
HSV	herpes simplex virus
ICP	intracranial pressure
ICU	intensive care unit
Ig	immunoglobulin
IM	intramuscular(ly)

INR	international normalized ratio
ISS	injury severity score
IUCD	intrauterine contraceptive device
IV	intravenous(ly)
J	joules
K^+	potassium
kg	kilogram
kph	kilometre per hour
KUB	kidneys, ureters, and bladder
L	litre
LAD	left anterior descending
LBBB	left bundle branch block
LCX	left circumflex artery
LDH	lactate dehydrogenase
m	metre
MERIT	mobile emergency response incident team
mg	milligram
min	minute
mL	millilitre
mm	millimetre
mmol	millimol
MMR	measles, mumps, rubella
mph	miles per hour
MRI	magnetic resonance imaging
MRSA	meticillin-resistant *Staphylococcus aureus*
mU	milli-units
N_2O	nitrous oxide
Na^+	sodium
NAC	*N*-acetyl cysteine
NAPQI	*N*-acetyl-p-benzoquinoneimine
ng	nanogram
NHS	National Health Service
NICE	National Institute for Health and Clinical Excellence
NPIS	National Poisons Information Service
NSAID	non-steroidal anti-inflammatory drug
NSTEMI	non-ST-elevation myocardial infarction
O_2	oxygen
OHEM	*Oxford Handbook of Emergency Medicine*

O&G	obstetrics and gynaecology
PCI	percutaneous coronary intervention
pCO_2	partial pressure of carbon dioxide
PEA	pulseless electrical activity
PEF(R)	peak expiratory flow (rate)
PEP	post-exposure prophylaxis
pH	power of hydrogen
pO_2	partial pressure of oxygen
POP	plaster of Paris
PSVT	paroxysmal supraventricular tachycardia
PV	per vagina
RBC	red blood cell
RCA	right coronary artery
Rh	rhesus
RNA	ribonucleic acid
RSI	rapid sequence intubation
RSV	respiratory syncytial virus
s	seconds
SaO_2	arterial oxygen saturation
SBA	single best answer
SBAR	situation, background, assessment, recommendation
SCIWORA	Spinal cord injury without radiological abnormality
SIRS	systemic inflammatory response syndrome
spp.	species
STI	sexually transmitted infection
SVT	supraventricular tachycardia
TIA	transient ischaemic attack
TIMI	Thrombolysis in Myocardial Infarction (risk score)
TSS	toxic shock syndrome
U	unit
UK	United Kingdom
UTI	urinary tract infection
V	volts
VA	visual acuity
VF	ventricular fibrillation
VT	ventricular tachycardia
WBC	white blood (cell) count
WHO	World Health Organization

HOW TO USE THIS BOOK

Oxford Assess and Progress, Emergency Medicine has been carefully designed to ensure you get the most out of your revision. Here is a brief guide to some of the features and learning tools.

Organization of content

Chapter editorials will help you unpick tricky subjects, and when it's late at night and you need something to remind you why you're doing this, you'll find words of encouragement!

Single Best Answer (SBAs) questions are indicated with this symbol 💡 and Extended Matching Questions (EMQs) 💡. Answers can be found at the end of each chapter. First the SBA answers 🖐, and then the EMQ answers 🖐.

How to read an answer

Unlike other revision guides on the market, this one is full of feedback, so you should understand exactly why each answer is correct.

With every answer there is an explanation of why that particular choice is the most appropriate. For some questions there is additional explanation of why the distracters are less suitable. Where relevant you will also be directed to sources of further information, such as the *Oxford Handbook of Emergency Medicine* (OHEM), websites, and journal articles. →http://www.institute.nhs.uk

Progression points

The questions in every chapter are ordered by level of difficulty and competence, indicated by the following symbols:

★ *Graduate 'should know'* – you should be aiming to get all of these correct.

★ ★ *Graduate 'nice to know'* – these are a bit tougher but not above your capabilities!

★ ★ ★   *Foundation Doctor 'should know'* – these will really test your understanding.

★ ★ ★ ★   *Foundation Doctor 'nice to know'* – give these a go when you're ready to challenge yourself!

Oxford Handbook of Emergency Medicine

The OHEM page references are given with the answers to some questions. OHEM 4th edn → p402 Please note that this reference is to the fourth edition of the OHEM, and that subsequent editions are unlikely to have the same material in exactly the same place.

The Online Resource Centre

Bonus questions will be released monthly in the run up to final medical examinations.

   www.oxfordtextbooks.co.uk/orc/gupta/

CHAPTER 1
GENERAL APPROACH

'It is not a case we are treating; it is a living, palpitating, alas, too often suffering fellow creature.'

John Brown

This chapter will focus on the day-to-day issues encountered in the ED for an overall understanding of the scenarios new doctors are expected to face on the very first day of their exciting career.

The first issue dealt with in this chapter is triage. Triage is the hub of clinical practice and used on a regular basis in one form or another. Although some departments have gradually developed the service of 'see and treat' and escaping triage, it is still applied formally or informally by a practising clinician. It is vital to prioritize patients attending with a wide range of clinical presentations. A few questions on this topic are included to give a flavour of what to expect when you join the ED.

The other issue discussed in this chapter is legal medicine, which again a newly qualified doctor may encounter on their first entry to the ED. But, it must be emphasized that plenty of support is provided to newcomers to put them at ease so that they may use their initial few days for settling into the department. To overcome the dilemma of ethical and legal issues, doctors can also contact medical defence organizations (the Medical Defence Union, the Medical Protection Society, etc.) and almost every doctor subscribes to one of the unions for this kind of support.

It is increasingly recognized that an appropriate level of communication is of the utmost importance for the safer and effective care of patients attending the ED. There is always the issue of when to refer a borderline case to a specialty peer for possible admission and further care. I am sure there are innumerable examples of a junior doctor feeling pressured to send a patient home inappropriately. Therefore the system of SBAR has been included in this chapter to remind every junior doctor as to how best to make effective referrals, no matter at what stage of their career they are or the clinical setting in which they work.

Lastly, dealing with a situation involving a major incident or disaster is always at the heart of every ED. Although such situations are primarily the responsibility of the senior clinicians and nursing staff, junior doctors—who are integral members of the team—are equally involved in the successful management of a potentially overwhelming situation. ■

GENERAL APPROACH
SINGLE BEST ANSWERS

1. A 75-year-old man has been resuscitated for 45min following a cardiac arrest. There is no sign of return of the circulation and a decision has been made to stop resuscitation. His relatives are waiting and are unaware of the decision. Which is the *single* most appropriate step to take? ★

A Bringing the relatives into the resuscitation room to break the news to them

B Sending an FY1 doctor to break the news

C Sending a nurse to reassure them that the team is still trying its best

D Sending a senior nurse to break the news in the waiting room

E The team leader and a nurse meeting the relatives in the relatives' room to break the news

2. A 20-year-old man has bruises and abrasions on his arms and hands following a fall after consuming 10 cans of lager. At the initial assessment in the ED, his heart rate is 70bpm, BP 110/68 mmHg, respiratory rate 20breaths/min, bedside capillary blood glucose 5.2mmol/L, and his GCS score is 15/15. While waiting to be seen he has started shouting, using abusive language towards the assessment nurse. Which is the *single* most appropriate next step? ★

A Arranging for a blood alcohol level

B Calling the security

C Ignoring the patient until he calms down

D Restraining him physically

E Using emergency sedation

3. A 28-year-old man has been brought to the ED in an ambulance after being involved in a road traffic collision. He is unconscious and is being resuscitated by the trauma team. The police officer requests a blood sample to check his alcohol level. Which is the *single* most appropriate step to take? ★

A Asking for the forensic medical examiner to collect the sample

B Refusing the request

C Taking a blood sample and hand it over to the police

D Taking a blood sample to send to the hospital lab

E Waiting until the patient wakes up to obtain consent

4. A 35-year-old woman has twisted her right ankle while walking her dog. She has swelling and severe pain on the outer aspect of the ankle and can partially weightbear. She has already been given analgesia. Which is the *single* most appropriate triage category she should be in? ★

A Category 1 (immediate)

B Category 2 (very urgent)

C Category 3 (urgent)

D Category 4 (standard)

E Category 5 (non-urgent)

5. A 78-year-old man has had abdominal pain for 6h. He has vomited three times and has not opened his bowels since yesterday. His pulse is 90bpm, BP 140/85mmHg, and respiratory rate 20breathes/min. His pain score is 6/10. Which is the *single* most appropriate triage category for him? ★

A Category 1 (immediate)

B Category 2 (very urgent)

C Category 3 (urgent)

D Category 4 (standard)

E Category 5 (non-urgent)

6. A 46-year-old unconscious woman is being brought to the ED by blue light ambulance. According to the paramedics she had a severe headache, which started suddenly about 6h ago. Her heart rate is 50bpm and BP 150/80mmHg. Which is her *single* most appropriate triage category? ★

A Category 1 (immediate)

B Category 2 (very urgent)

C Category 3 (urgent)

D Category 4 (standard)

E Category 5 (non-urgent)

7. An 82-year-old man is brought in with sudden onset of pain in his upper abdomen, which is radiating to his back. He is feeling dizzy and unwell and he is sweaty and pale. His pulse is 100bpm and BP 120/80mmHg. He has tenderness in the upper abdomen with palpable pulsation. Suspecting a case of ruptured AAA, a referral is made over the phone to the surgical registrar but this is refused without seeing the patient. The registrar also advises to send the patient home after managing him with analgesia as he feels it does not seem like a ruptured AAA. Which is the *single* most appropriate next step in his management? ★★★★

A Calling the on-call surgical consultant

B Continuing to negotiate with the registrar to accept the referral

C Discharging the patient after giving him analgesia as advised

D Reporting the registrar to the medical director

E Seeking help from senior ED staff

8. A 65-year-old man has had acute retention of urine for 4h and has lower abdominal pain. A final year medical student wishes to catheterize the patient as she has undergone training on a plastic model on several occasions. The department is busy. Which is the *single* most appropriate step to take? ★ ★ ★

A Allowing her to catheterize on her own, provided the patient has given consent

B Allowing her to catheterize under supervision of an experienced doctor

C Instructing her to learn this procedure after she has qualified

D Postponing the training as the department is very busy

E Refusing her request as the patient is in pain

9. A 55-year-old man with a history of longstanding alcohol misuse and living rough has been pronounced dead in the ED after prolonged resuscitation. He had attended the ED a month earlier and a GP a couple of days before. Which one is the *single* reason to report his death to a coroner or Procurator Fiscal (in Scotland)? ★ ★ ★

A Alcohol misuse

B Death in ED

C Earlier ED attendance

D GP visit

E Living rough

10. A high-speed train has derailed at a nearby station. The ED receives a phone call that it is about to receive 27 patients with various grades of injuries; four of them died at the scene of the accident. The department is very busy and already has 48 patients. Which is the *single* most appropriate next step? ★ ★ ★ ★

A Booking the accident victims in at the reception as normal

B Discharging all the 48 patients in the department to create space

C Dispatching a MERIT to assist at the scene

D Doctors and nurses should follow their action cards

E Informing the ambulance service not to bring these trauma patients to your ED as the department is very busy

ANSWERS

Single Best Answers

1. E ★   OHEM, 4th edn →pp24–5

Make sure that if you are the person breaking the news, a link nurse is with you. Confirm that you have the correct patient details and check who the relatives are. Meet them in the relatives' room and sensitively break the news, clearly informing them that their loved one is dead. Offer them the opportunity to see the body as soon as possible. Don't call them in the middle of resuscitation without adequate support, i.e. a senior nurse, to explain to them what is happening.

It is the team leader's duty, who is usually a consultant, registrar-level trainee, or a specialist trainee year three and above, to meet the relatives. An FY1 should not be asked to do this in the early stage of their career, rather they might accompany the team leader to have a learning experience.

Towards the end of conversation, offer the relatives additional support by asking, 'Is there anything I can do?' (e.g. further clarification, contacting other relatives, getting a cup of tea or coffee).

2. B ★   OHEM, 4th edn →pp628–9

You need to get help by calling security or the police; safety of the staff and others is the first priority.

A: It is not routine practice to request for blood alcohol level, moreover, it is unsafe and dangerous to try to take blood from such a patient.

C: It is important that the patient does not distress the other patients and relatives in the waiting room, and ignoring him may cause further unrest in the area.

D: Restraining by staff is never advisable as it requires special training and authority. Some security guards in the ED may not have power to or even training for restraining. If the situation worsens and the patient requires restraining, the police may be called.

E: Injectable emergency sedation is not safe and should only be undertaken by senior experienced staff if needed.

N.B. It must be recognized that the patient's aggressive behaviour may be because of a treatable acute medical condition such as acute hypoglycaemia, acute hypoxia, acute retention of urine or head injury (in this case). The consumption of alcohol may complicate the situation further or may result in such emergencies. Therefore, it is important to first exclude such emergencies.

→ http://www.nice.org.uk/nicemedia/live/10964/29716/29716.pdf

3. A ★   OHEM, 4th edn →p30

According to the Police Reform Act 2002, the police can request a blood sample from an unconscious patient, which is only to be collected by a forensic medical examiner (police surgeon), to be tested later depending on the patient giving consent.

4. D ★   OHEM, 4th edn →p7

Triage is done in the ED so that life-threatening emergencies are seen first. The most commonly used tool is the National Triage Scale. Cases such as cardiac arrests are category 1. Category 2 patients are supposed to be seen by a doctor within 5–10min. Category 3, 4, and 5 patients should be seen within 1, 2, and 4h, respectively. This patient in question should be placed in the standard category, i.e. should be seen in within 2h as she has significant pain and swelling. Though many EDs may not triage patients with minor ailments and such cases may be seen directly in the minor/walk-in part of the department, it is important to have some basic knowledge about the triage system.

5. C ★   OHEM, 4th edn →p7

This patient has moderate pain in the abdomen with tachycardia, but is not shocked. So it is safe at this time for him to wait for 1h to be seen by a doctor.

6. A ★   OHEM, 4th edn →p7

This patient is unconscious and her airway is compromised, therefore, she requires immediate airway protection.

7. E ★★★★   OHEM, 4th edn →p9

A patient with suspected ruptured AAA requires inpatient investigation and treatment. Referral of patients in the ED is often made by telephone, which may create problems at times.

However, do pause and reflect on the appropriateness of the referral before bleeping a specialist. When referring give a clear and concise summary of the history, examination findings, investigations, and treatment. Make clear at the outset of the conversation that the referral is a request for a specialist opinion.

The easily memorized communication system of SBAR may be used during conversations about patients, especially critical ones, requiring a clinician's immediate attention and action. This method may be followed in any clinical situation, e.g. inpatient, outpatient, urgent or non-urgent referrals. The SBAR is summarized below.

S	Situation	<ul><li>Identify yourself/the site or unit you are calling from</li><li>Identify the patient by name and give the reason for your report</li><li>Describe your concern</li></ul>
B	Background	<ul><li>Give the patient's reason for admission</li><li>Explain significant medical history</li><li>Give the patient's background: admission diagnosis, lab results, diagnostic results etc.</li></ul>
A	Assessment	<ul><li>Patient's vital signs</li><li>Contraction pattern</li><li>Clinical impression and concerns</li></ul>
R	Recommendation	<ul><li>Explain what you need – be specific about request and timeframe</li><li>Make suggestions</li><li>Clarify expectations</li></ul>

© NHS Institute for Innovation and Improvement, 2008.

If as a junior doctor you think a patient requires admission and, for whatever reason, this is declined, it is inadvisable to become aggressive or rude, but instead contact the senior ED medical staff to the speak to the specialist team.

A: The ED consultant may contact the surgical consultant if required.

B: This may be an option if the patient is stable and there is time on hand to negotiate. In cases of a ruptured AAA, the patient may deteriorate rapidly, therefore, involving senior ED medical staff would be time-saving and an appropriate action.

C: Do not discharge such patients if you are not happy and suspect serious illness that requires inpatient treatment.

D: It is inappropriate for an FY1 to refer another doctor to the medical director. Such decisions should be left to the ED consultants to consider.

→ http://www.institute.nhs.uk/. Search 'SBAR'.

8. B ★ ★ ★ OHEM, 4th edn →p15

The patient has acute urinary retention. Provided they have given consent, the student should be encouraged to learn the procedure live under supervision of a senior medical member of staff.
The student should know the method from her previous practice on the manikin.

A: Do not allow her to perform the procedure for the first time unsupervised as male catheterization may be a difficult procedure.

C: This is not appropriate as the student needs real life practical experience where possible.

D: The ED is almost always busy. Hands-on training should be provided among all other service activities.

E: Patients with acute urinary retention are almost always in pain. Therefore, it is not appropriate reason for refusal. The only time the student may not perform the procedure would be if the patient refuses to give consent.

9. B ★ ★ ★ OHEM, 4th edn →p26

All ED deaths are required to be reported to a coroner.
Any suspicious death must be immediately reported to the police/coroner or Procurator Fiscal (in Scotland). Coroners must also be informed of deaths if related to an accident, suicide, employment, or recent detention in police or prison custody.

A. The patient has a long-term illness, which might have caused his death, so there is no need to report for this reason.

C: If the certifying doctor has not seen the deceased after the death or within 14 days before the death it should be reported to a coroner. Therefore, earlier ED attendance a month ago may not be the indication of referring to the coroner.

D and E: These are not reasons for reporting deaths to a coroner.

A coroner is a doctor or lawyer responsible for investigating deaths in particular situations; they can also arrange for a post-mortem examination of the body, if necessary. An inquest is a legal inquiry into the causes and circumstances of a death. If death occurs in any of the following circumstances, the attending doctor may report it to a coroner:

- After an accident or injury
- Following an industrial disease
- During a surgical operation
- Before recovery from anaesthesia
- If the cause of death is unknown
- If the death was violent or unnatural, for example, suicide, accident, or drug or alcohol overdose
- If the death was sudden and unexplained, for instance, sudden infant death (cot death).

Anyone who is concerned about the cause of a death can inform a coroner about it, but in most cases a death will be reported to the coroner by a doctor or the police.

→ http://www.direct.gov.uk/en/governmentcitizensandrights/death/whattodoafteradeath/dg_066713

10. D ★ ★ ★ ★ OHEM, 4th edn →pp38–9

A major incident is a special arrangement that is made by health services to receive live casualties depending on their number, severity, type, or location. Every hospital receiving emergencies must have a major incident plan to use when normal resources are unable to cope and special arrangements are needed. The plan usually has actions cards, which state in bullet points what action an FY1, FY2, specialist trainee or consultant should take during such an event. As soon as information is received from ambulance control that a major incident has been 'DECLARED' the department should start preparing to receive the casualties and all the doctors and nurses should check their action cards to know their roles.

A: All the patients arriving from the incident should be labelled with a unique major incident number, which is used in all notes, forms, blood samples, etc. A number of receptionists will follow the patients to collect their names and addresses as soon as possible.

B: Only the less serious patients or minor injury patients may be referred to an alternative healthcare team, e.g. GPs. Seriously ill patients may be transferred to special ward areas as specified in the major incident plan. Medical patients may be sent to medical wards to be seen by the medical teams directly.

C: A MERIT (previously called Mobile Medical Team) should be sent from a nearby supporting hospital that is not receiving the casualties of the major incident.

E: The decision to receive the patients from a major incident is made by the senior officials at ambulance control or police service and not a hospital.

→ http://www.dh.gov.uk/prod_consum_dh/groups/dh_digitalassets/@dh/@en/@ps/documents/digitalasset/dh_114467.pdf

CHAPTER 2

LIFE-THREATENING EMERGENCIES

'Don't take your organs to heaven with you. Heaven knows we need them here.'

Anon

When a '43-year-old male with a cardiac arrest' or a '63-year-old hypotensive with tachycardia and shortness of breath' message flies through the red phone from the ambulance control, it is normal for junior doctors to get a bit apprehensive in the first few days of their clinical life. However, knowledge of and following the few basic steps for a rapid assessment and management of the airway, breathing, circulation, disability, and exposure (ABCDE) that are discussed in this chapter may alleviate some of their nervousness and give them the requisite confidence to face such life-threatening emergencies with energy and vigour.

The routine practice of taking a history and performing a physical examination, followed by investigations and treatment, is not applicable in emergency situations as time is of the essence. Brief assessment is followed by treatment. A brief history may be collected from the paramedics as often the patient is not in a condition to talk. In the event of a cardiac arrest, protocols are always available in almost all the EDs in the UK and you should follow these. In today's training climate, a new FY1 will never be left on his or her own to face a situation which is beyond their competence. Help is always available in the form of senior doctors, nurses, and other staff.

It is important to first manage the basic ABCDE and, then not missing any of the simple clinical observations such as respiratory rate, capillary refill time, and capillary blood glucose testing. A short but succinct systematic physical examination is important for nailing the main problems and treating them immediately. Most of the time, the underlying cause of acute symptoms is obvious from the outset; at other times, you may need to request some additional tests later to establish the diagnosis. Sticking to ABCDE in the first instance will support the patient and buy time, allowing the doctor to get to the root of the problem, and do what is necessary to help the patient.

This chapter has scenarios relating to life-threatening clinical presentations such as anaphylaxis and hoarseness to help ascertain the diagnosis and initiate appropriate treatment immediately. In cases of cardiac arrest, various situations have been included—almost all of them based on real life—to give a flavour of how to approach and start treatment, thereby maintaining a smooth transition for the patient between care provided by the prehospital team and the ED. ■

LIFE-THREATENING EMERGENCIES
SINGLE BEST ANSWERS

1. A 28-year-old woman has suddenly developed a red rash all over the body following a wasp sting. Her pulse is 100bpm, BP 120/70mmHg, and respiratory rate 24breaths/min. Which *single* most important clinical feature is indicative for adrenaline (epinephrine) treatment? ★

A Diarrhoea

B Hoarseness of voice

C Rhinitis

D Swelling of lip

E Wheals

2. A 28-year-old woman has suddenly developed a red itchy rash with wheals all over her body. Her lips are swollen and she has noisy breathing. Her pulse is 124bpm, BP 90/70mmHg, and respiratory rate 30breaths/min. Which is the *single* most appropriate immediate treatment? ★

A Adrenaline (epinephrine) 0.5mL (mg) 1 in 100 IM

B Adrenaline (epinephrine) 0.5mL (mg) 1 in 1000 IM

C Adrenaline (epinephrine) 0.5mL (mg) 1 in 10 000 IM

D Adrenaline (epinephrine) 0.5mL (mg) 1 in 100 000 IM

E Adrenaline (epinephrine) 0.5mL (mg) 1 in 1 000 000 IM

3. A 22-year-old woman has suddenly developed a red itchy rash with wheals all over her body after a meal. Her pulse is 80bpm, BP 110/70mmHg, and respiratory rate is 22breaths/min. Her oxygen saturation is 99% on oxygen. Which is the *single* most appropriate immediate treatment? ★

A Adrenaline (epinephrine)

B Chlorphenamine

C Hydrocortisone

D Normal saline

E Salbutamol

4. A 32-year-old man with known allergy to peanuts has suddenly developed a red itchy rash with wheals all over his body after a meal. His mouth and tongue are swollen. His pulse is 130bpm, BP 80/60mmHg, and respiratory rate 30breaths/min with audible stridor. Which is the *single* most likely underlying immunological reaction? ★

A Type I

B Type II

C Type III

D Type IV

E Type V

5. A 22-year-old woman, who is known to have peanut allergy, has suddenly developed a red itchy rash with wheals all over her body after a meal. Her pulse is 80bpm, BP 110/70mmHg, and respiratory rate 22breaths/min. Her oxygen saturation is 99% on oxygen. After receiving treatment her rashes have started to disappear and she is feeling better. Which is the *single* most appropriate discharge option? ★

A Advising her to see GP and collect prescriptions for antihistamines

B Discharging her with steroids after 24h observation

C Giving an antihistamine and make a follow-up appointment with a specialist

D Giving an antihistamine and steroids to take home after 4h observation

E Prescribing an adrenaline (epinephrine) auto-injector and antihistamines

6. A 38-year-old woman has suddenly developed a red itchy rash with wheals all over her body after her evening meal. Her lips are swollen and she has noisy breathing. Her pulse is 120bpm, BP 90/70mmHg, and respiratory rate 30breaths/min. After initial treatment with adrenaline (epinephrine) and IV saline infusion, the clinical parameters are: the pulse 100bpm, BP 110/80mmHg, and respiratory rate 25breaths/min. Which is the *single* most appropriate next management? ★

A Admitting to a ward for observation and further treatment

B Discharging her with an antihistamine and steroids

C Discharging her with an urgent follow-up to see an allergy specialist

D Not discharging until the patient is seen by an allergy specialist on the wards

E Observing her for a couple of hours in the ED

7. A 58-year-old man is receiving CPR in the ED. After delivery of two shocks the heart rhythm at the end of the second cycle is as shown in Fig. 2.1.

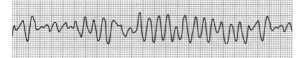

Which is the *single* most appropriate next action? ★ ★ ★

A Administering amiodarone

B Administering both adrenaline (epinephrine) and amiodarone

C Checking the pulse

D Giving a third shock

E Resuming chest compressions

8. A 62-year-old man is receiving CPR. He has been given two shocks. At the end of the second cycle the monitor shows an unchanged rhythm (Fig. 2.2).

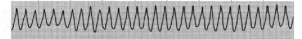

Which is the *single* most appropriate immediate next action? ★ ★ ★

A Applying precordial thump

B Giving fourth shock

C Giving IV amiodarone

D Giving second dose of adrenaline

E Resume chest compressions

9. A 67-year-old man has had chest pain for 2h. While being monitored in the resuscitation room, he collapses and loses consciousness. His rhythm is shown in Fig. 2.3.

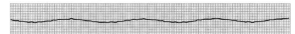

Which is the *single* most appropriate next immediate action? ★

A Checking oxygen connections

B Commencing CPR

C Feeling for carotid pulse

D Giving IV atropine

E Measuring BP

10. A 64-year-old man has attended the ED with central chest pain. While being monitored in the resuscitation room, he started feeling unwell. He is delivered a shock under short-acting anaesthesia. His rhythm is shown in Fig. 2.4.

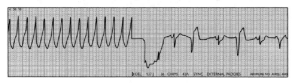

Which is the *single* most appropriate next immediate action? ★

A Checking breathing

B Checking connections to monitor

C Feeling carotid pulse

D Measuring BP

E Performing 12-lead electrocardiogram

11. A 53-year-old man is receiving CPR in the ED. Immediately after delivery of the first shock his heart rhythm on the monitor is as shown in Fig. 2.5.

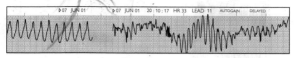

Which is the *single* most appropriate next action? ★ ★ ★

A Checking breathing

B Checking pulse

C Giving a second shock

D Giving adrenaline (epinephrine)

E Resuming chest compressions

12. A 48-year-old woman who has been coughing for the last 3 days is now very short of breath. Her heart rate is 110bpm, BP 110/60mmHg, respiratory rate 35breaths/min, and temperature 38.5°C. Her chest X-ray shows consolidation in the right mid zone. Her lactate is 2mmol/L and PaO_2 is 8.5kPa on air. Which is the *single* most appropriate severity of illness she has? ★ ★

A Multiple organ failure

B Sepsis

C Septic shock

D Severe sepsis

E SIRS

13. A 47-year-old woman who has been having lower abdominal pain for the past 4 four days is now very unwell with rigors. Her temperature is 39.5°C, heart rate 120bpm, BP 80/55mmHg, respiratory rate 30breaths/min. Her serum lactate is 4.3mmol/L and WBC 14×10⁹/L. Which is the *single* most appropriate initial fluid therapy? ★ ★

A 0.5L of colloid in 2h

B 1L of Hartmann's solution in 2h

C 1L of normal saline in half an hour

D 2 units of blood in 2h

E Fluid under central venous pressure guidance

14. A 49-year-old woman who has had dysuria for 3 days is now very unwell with rigors and pain in the loins. Her temperature is 39.0°C, heart rate 110bpm, BP 80/55mmHg, and respiratory rate 32breaths/min. Her serum lactate is 4.1mmol/L and WBC 13×10⁹/L. She has been given oxygen and a fluid challenge. A urinary catheter and central line is being inserted. Which is the *single* most important goal to achieve with further fluid management? ★ ★

A Body temperature ≤37.5°C

B Central venous pressure of ≥8mmHg

C Serum lactate <3mmol/L

D Systolic BP of ≥90mmHg

E Urine output ≥1mL/h/kg body weight

15. A 45-year-old man who has been coughing for 3 days is now short of breath. His temperature is 38.5°C, heart rate 110bpm, BP 110/60mmHg, and respiratory rate 35breaths/min. Which is the *single* most appropriate severity of illness he has? ★ ★

A Multiple organ failure

B Sepsis

C Septic shock

D Severe sepsis

E SIRS

LIFE-THREATENING EMERGENCIES
EXTENDED MATCHING QUESTIONS

Management of cardiac arrest

For each of the following cases, choose the *single* most appropriate next action from the list of options below. Each answer may be used once, more than once, or not at all.

A Adrenaline (epinephrine)

B Amiodarone

C Atropine

D Check breathing

E Check monitor

F Check pulse

G Check rhythm

H CPR

I Shock

J Synchronized cardioversion

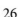

1. A 72-year-old man admitted with chest pain has collapsed suddenly in the resuscitation room while being monitored. CPR has been started and he has received a dose of adrenaline but his rhythm remains unchanged (Fig. 2.6).

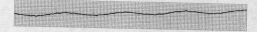

2. A 56-year-old man is receiving CPR. He has been given a first shock and 2min later, his rhythm is as shown in Fig. 2.7. Chest compression is started.

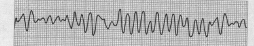

3. A 58-year-old man is having CPR. After receiving a shock and 2min of CPR his rhythm is as shown in Fig. 2.8.

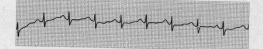

4. A 48-year-old man attends the ED with severe chest pain and shortness of breath. He collapses on the resuscitation trolley. He is unconscious, has no pulse and has the rhythm shown in Fig. 2.9. The chest compression is resumed.

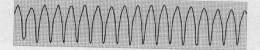

5. A 69-year-old woman is in cardiac arrest. She has received CPR for 2min and a dose of adrenaline (epinephrine) but the rhythm shown in Fig. 2.10 persists.

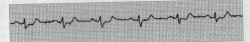

ANSWERS

Single Best Answers

1. B ★   OHEM, 4th edn →p43

Adrenaline (epinephrine) is indicated in patients in shock or with airway compromise. Hoarseness (or stridor) is an indicator of potential airway obstruction; therefore, immediate IM adrenaline should be given. The other features listed are not life-threatening and should be treated with an antihistamine. This patient is not in shock. Patients with swelling of lips only do not require drug treatment but should be kept under close observation for potential respiratory obstruction, i.e. swelling extending into mouth, tongue, oropharynx, etc.

For UK resuscitation guidelines see Appendix 1.

→ www.resus.org.uk/

2. B ★   OHEM, 4th edn →p43

The correct dosage of adrenaline (epinephrine) is 0.5mL (mg) of 1:1000 IM, to be given when the patient is in shock, airway swelling or respiratory difficulty. IV adrenaline 1:10 000 or 1:100 000 slow IV may be given when patient has an immediate life-threatening condition or is in profound shock and its use is reserved for experienced clinicians. See Appendix 1.

→ www.resus.org.uk/

3. B ★   OHEM, 4th edn →p42

This is a common presentation in the ED of an acute urticarial reaction. Acute urticaria may be an IgE-mediated hypersensitivity reaction, similar to anaphylaxis. A variety of chemicals (e.g. foods, drugs) and physical stimuli (heat, wet, cold) may cause a similar type of reaction. There are other mechanisms also, namely complement, bradykinin, and substance P mediated reactions, and direct mast cell stimulation.

It is important to note that the urticaria may be a presentation of other underlying diseases. While managing such cases, take care to rule out any haemodynamic instability or potential airway obstruction, which should be dealt with first.

- Antihistamines are the first-line drugs in acute urticarial reactions, which work by blocking the H_1 and H_2 receptors present in the skin; 85% are H_1 and 15% are H_2 in the skin.
- Adrenaline (epinephrine) must only be considered in cases of haemodynamic instability or potential airway obstruction.
- Hydrocortisone takes 4–6h to act, so is of little benefit in acute stages. Systemic steroids are indicated to avoid the biphasic reactions in anaphylaxis.
- This patient is not in shock, therefore, may be observed closely with an IV line set up to start fluid if they deteriorate haemodynamically.
- Salbutamol nebulizer is indicated in presence of bronchospasm unresponsive to adrenaline.

See Appendix 1.

→ www.resus.org.uk/

4. A ★

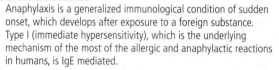

Anaphylaxis is a generalized immunological condition of sudden onset, which develops after exposure to a foreign substance. Type I (immediate hypersensitivity), which is the underlying mechanism of the most of the allergic and anaphylactic reactions in humans, is IgE mediated.

B: Type II reaction is an IgG- and IgM-mediated reaction (cytotoxic) and may also be involved in anaphylactoid reactions (anaphylaxis not produced by IgE-mediated reaction is called anaphylactoid reaction).

C: Type III reactions are immune complex, IgG, or IgM mediated. Anaphylactic reactions related to blood transfusion are caused by the overlapping type II and III reactions.

D: Type IV is T cell mediated and is not involved in the pathogenesis of anaphylaxis.

E: Type V is a part of the type II reaction, mediated by IgG or IgM (complement). Certain autoimmune diseases, such as myasthenia gravis and Graves' disease fall in this category. These are not related to anaphylaxis.

See Appendix 1.

→ www.resus.org.uk/

5. D ★

This is a common presentation in the ED of acute urticarial reaction. The patient may be discharged after being reviewed by a senior clinician 4–6h later if showing signs of continuous improvement. She should be prescribed oral steroids and antihistamines for 3 days. There is no requirement for 24h observation, which is only indicated in severe anaphylactic reactions. The patient is already known to have peanut allergy, so immediate referral to an allergy clinic may not be required, unless she does not have a treatment plan. The referral may be done later by her GP. However, a reminder to avoid trigger food would be helpful. Adrenaline (epinephrine) auto-injectors are given to patients who are at increased risk of an idiopathic anaphylactic reaction, or for anyone at continued high risk of reaction. They should not be given to patients directly by the ED without consulting a specialist. There is not much point in sending the patient to her GP for collection of a prescription as it may cause delay in receiving treatment. See Appendix 1.

→ www.resus.org.uk/

6. A ★

The patient should be admitted for at least 6h and must be discharged only after being assessed by a senior clinician. They may need further treatment. In some circumstances patients may require admission for 24h. This caution is particularly applicable to:

- Severe idiopathic anaphylactic reactions
- If patient has severe asthma following reaction
- Reactions with the possibility of continuing absorption of allergen (as in this patient)
- Patients with past history of biphasic reactions
- Patients presenting in the evening or night.

See Appendix 1.

→ http://www.resus.org.uk/pages/reaction.pdf

7. E ★★★   OHEM, 4th edn →p55

The rhythm is VF. The first cycle begins with delivery of a shock followed by 2min of CPR. At the beginning of the second cycle, check the rhythm. If it remains in VF, deliver a second shock and continue CPR. Make sure chest compression continues when the defibrillator is charged. The chest compression is to be delivered at the rate of 100-120 times per minute with compression depth of 5-6 cm (in adults). Refer to the UK resuscitation guidelines (2010) for the flow chart (also shown in Appendix 2 (BLS) and

Appendix 3 (ALS)). The sequence of management is described in Fig. 2.11 below.

→ www.resus.org.uk/pages/als.pdf

Treatment of shockable rhythms (VF/VT)

1. Confirm cardiac arrest—check for signs of life or if trained to do so, breathing and pulse simultaneously.
2. Call resuscitation team.
3. Perform uninterrupted chest compressions while applying self-adhesive defibrillation/monitoring pads—one below the right clavicle and the other in the V6 position in the mid-axillary line.
4. Plan actions before pausing CPR for rhythm analysis and communicate these to the team.
5. Stop chest compressions; confirm VF from the ECG.
6. Resume chest compressions immediately; simultaneously, the designated person selects the appropriate energy on the defibrillator (150–200 J biphasic for the first shock and 150–360 J biphasic for subsequent shocks) and presses the charge button.
7. While the defibrillator is charging, warn all rescuers other than the individual performing the chest compressions to 'stand clear' and remove any oxygen delivery device as appropriate. Ensure that the rescuer giving the compressions is the only person touching the patient.
8. Once the defibrillator is charged, tell the rescuer doing the chest compressions to 'stand clear' ; when clear, give the shock.
9. Without reassessing the rhythm or feeling for a pulse, restart CPR using a ratio of 30:2, starting with chest compressions.
10. Continue CPR for 2 min; the team leader prepares the team for the next pause in CPR.
11. Pause briefly to check the monitor.
12. If VF/VT, repeat steps 6–11 above and deliver a second shock.
13. If VF/VT persists repeat steps 6–8 above and deliver a third shock. Resume chest compressions immediately and then give adrenaline 1 mg IV and amiodarone 300 mg IV while performing a further 2 min CPR.
14. Repeat this 2 min CPR—rhythm/pulse check—defibrillation sequence if VF/VT persists.
15. Give further adrenaline 1 mg IV after alternate shocks (i.e., approximately every 3–5 min).

If organised electrical activity compatible with a cardiac output is seen during a rhythm check, seek evidence of return of spontaneous circulation (ROSC):

- Check a central pulse and end-tidal CO_2 trace if available
- If there is evidence of ROSC, start post-resuscitation care.
- If no signs of ROSC, continue CPR and switch to the non-shockable algorithm.

8. E ★ ★ ★   OHEM, 4th edn →p55

The rhythm is VT. In the absence of ROSC, the third cycle begins
with the delivery of a shock followed by 2min of chest compression.
Then give adrenaline and amiodarone IV. Refer to Fig. 2.11 for the
subsequent steps of resuscitation. See also Appendix 3 (ALS).

→ www.resus.org.uk/pages/als.pdf

9. C ★   OHEM, 4th edn →p53

This is an asystole arrest. Check the patient's pulse or other signs of
life to confirm the cardiac arrest and also check the connections of
the monitor quickly. If there is no pulse, commence CPR. Blood
pressure measurement is not a part of resuscitation unless there is a
palpable pulse. IV atropine is not recommended. See Appendix 8.

→ www.resus.org.uk/pages/inhresus.pdf

10. C ★

In the rhythm strip in Fig. 2.4, the first part is VT with
presence of palpable pulse. The patient was given synchronized
shock and as a result, the rhythm changed to sinus rhythm.
The next action is to check the central pulse, and/or signs
of life. If the pulse is present, then check the BP and perform
12-lead ECG. If the pulse is absent, start CPR, as the rhythm would
be PEA.

→ www.resus.org.uk/pages/als.pdf

11. E ★ ★ ★   OHEM, 4th edn →p55

The left side of the rhythm strip is VT. After the shock, the
rhythm changes to VF, followed by VT. The rhythm is unstable,
showing intermittently both these arrhythmias. The first cycle
begins with the delivery of a shock followed by 2min of CPR after
which the rhythm should be checked. At the beginning of the
second cycle, if he remains in VF or VT without change of
morphology, deliver a second shock and continue CPR. If there is
any change in the morphology of the rhythm, check the pulse
and/or signs of life at the end of the cycle.

→ www.resus.org.uk/pages/als.pdf

The patient has severe sepsis. The various septic conditions are given below:

SIRS: Any two or more out of tachycardia, (heart rate >90); tachypnoea, (respiratory rate >20); pyrexia (>38°C); hypothermia (<36°C) and WBC >12 or <4×10⁹/L.

Septic shock: refractory hypotension and organ dysfunction, mortality 40–70%.

Sepsis syndrome (severe sepsis): SIRS + documented source of infection + organ dysfunction. (This patient has a documented source of infection in the chest + organ dysfunction (CVS and respiratory) + SIRS); mortality 25–70%.

Sepsis = SIRS + confirmed infectious process.

→ http://chestjournal.chestpubs.org/content/101/6/1644.full.pdf±htm

The patient has septic shock, which requires immediate resuscitation by giving fluid challenge therapy. This is done by giving 1L of crystalloid or 300–500mL of colloid in 30min. Further fluid requirements are guided by the initial response. The fluid may be given immediately by peripheral IV line through a wide-bore cannula, but central line insertion may be required to monitor the central venous pressure, especially in the elderly with poor cardiovascular reserve.

This patient needs aggressive therapy with the help of intensivists. The goals of therapy are:

- Central venous pressure of 8–12mmHg
- Central venous or mixed venous saturation ≥65%
- Mean arterial BP ≥65mmHg
- Urine output ≥0.5mL/kg/h.

For further information, see the *Oxford Handbook of Acute Medicine*, 3rd edn, (pp316–19) and *Emergencies in Critical Care* (p118).

→ www.survivingsepsis.org/SiteCollectionDocuments/Final%2008%20SSC%20Guidelines.pdf

The patient has septic shock, which requires immediate resuscitation by giving fluid challenge therapy. This is done by giving 1L of crystalloid (20mL/kg of body weight) or 300–500mL of colloid in 30min. Further fluid requirements are guided by the initial response to achieve the following goals within the first 6h:

- Central venous pressure of ≥8–12mmHg
- Central venous saturation >65%
- Mean arterial BP >65mmHg
- Urine output 0.5mL/kg/h

For further information, see the *Oxford Handbook of Acute Medicine*, 3rd edn, (pp316–19).

→ www.survivingsepsis.org/SiteCollectionDocuments/Final%20 08%20SSC%20Guidelines.pdf

15. E ★ ★   OHEM, 4th edn → p61

The patient has SIRS. The various definitions are given in Answer 12. Mortality in sepsis is 7%.

→ http://chestjournal.chestpubs.org/content/101/6/1644.full. pdf±htm

Extended Matching Questions

1. H ★   OHEM, 4th edn → pp54–5

The patient is in asystole. The treatment for asystole is to start CPR and a dose of adrenaline (epinephrine) (1mg IV) See Appendix 3.

2. I ★   OHEM, 4th edn → pp52–5

The patient is in VF and should receive an immediate shock followed by CPR for 2min, then a rhythm check, which is still the same. He then should immediately receive another followed by another set of CPR for a further 2min.

3. F ★   OHEM, 4th edn → pp52–5

The patient was either in VF or pulseless VT, for which he received the shock. Immediately after delivering the shock, CPR should be continued for 2min followed by a rhythm check, which has changed to sinus. As it might be compatible with life, the next action is to *check the pulse*/seek evidence of ROSC.

4. I ★   OHEM, 4th edn → pp52–5

The patient has pulseless VT and the correct treatment in such situations is to deliver a shock (unsynchronized) (150–360J biphasic or 360J monophasic) without delay.

This patient has PEA. After the first cycle of a dose of adrenaline (epinephrine) and 2min of CPR, a rhythm check shows the same rhythm. CPR should be reinitiated. A further dose of adrenaline should only be given every 3–5min (every other cycle).

→ www.resus.org.uk/pages/als.pdf

CHAPTER 3
MEDICINE

'He's the best physician that knows the worthlessness of the most medicines.'

Benjamin Franklin

This chapter encompasses questions on acute and subacute clinical situations spread over the various branches of general medicine, which include cardiology, gastroenterology, respiratory system, etc. The questions cover common presentations and anyone who starts practising emergency medicine will encounter such cases right from the beginning. Some of these may be brought by blue light ambulance in an acute stage (acute hypoxia, acute asthma, acute exacerbation of COPD, GI haemorrhage, myocardial infarction, arrhythmias, and many others). Therefore, it is important to have a good grasp of the fundamentals of common ailments so that timely intervention can avoid development of life-threatening complications.

A variety of ECGs and chest X-rays have been included in this chapter to cover the common emergencies encountered in regular practice, both in the resuscitation room and in the trolley area. The aim is not necessarily to make you an expert in these areas, but to be able to recognize the patterns of important diseases in their acute stages, to expand your horizons further through seeing and treating more cases, by means of which vital confidence can be gained.

There is always an inclination that any patient presenting with chest pain has to have an ACS and the aim is to prove or disprove that it is so. Even after admission to a ward and further tests, the patient is often discharged without the reason of the chest pain being found out. So it is important to consider several other causes of chest pain. Once ACS becomes unlikely, pulmonary embolism should also be considered as an important differential.

With regard to the respiratory system, a severe or life-threatening asthma attack can be a daunting experience for the new doctor. Ask for help if you find the presentation is beyond your competence. In such a situation, you would need help from other specialties anyway. Timely intervention by an intensivist may save a young life. Anticipating airway obstruction in smoke inhalation is difficult most of the time, particularly when the patient appears to be talking normally, so it is important to recognize the importance of asking for senior help for further assessment.

The respiratory and cardiovascular systems have the advantage that the clinician can assess the patient with the help of a stethoscope, chest X-ray and ECGs, and so are probably a little less challenging than the GI system, where the symptoms are often vague to be able to reach a conclusive diagnosis. It is important to remember that in the ED, often an immediate diagnosis is not required to maintain a patient's stability. Sometimes, diagnosis establishment requires a battery of tests over a long period. However, it is important to try to differentiate between a surgical and medical abdomen at the very outset.

In the absence of special investigation modalities such as CT of the chest, echocardiography, endoscopy etc. in the ED, a patient with shortness of breath, wheeze, chest pain or GI bleed can be managed following the simple yet fundamental basic principles as described in this chapter. ■

SINGLE BEST ANSWERS

1. A 58-year-old man has had severe central chest pain for the last 5h. He is sweaty and unwell. His pulse is 120bpm, BP 140/90mmHg, and respiratory rate 30breaths/min. The ECG is shown in Fig. 3.1. (See the ECG suite at the back of the book for a larger version of this figure →p399.)

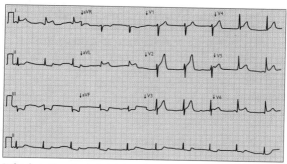

Which is the *single* initial underlying pathological event most likely to have caused this? ★

A Activation of platelet aggregation

B Blockage of coronary artery by thrombus

C Fissuring of an atheromatous plaque

D Previously critically impaired myocardial function

E Vasospasm induced by local inflammatory mediators

2. A 68-year-old man has had moderately severe chest pain for the last 5h. He is sweaty and unwell. His pulse is 120bpm, BP 140/90mmHg, and respiratory rate 25breaths/min. The ECG is shown in Fig. 3.2. (See the ECG suite at the back of the book for a larger version of this figure →p400.)

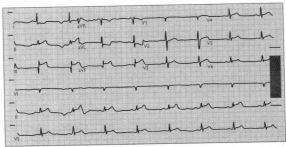

Which is the *single* area of the heart most likely to be involved? ★

A Anterior

B Anterolateral

C Anteroseptal

D Inferior

E Posterior

3. A 78-year-old man felt very unwell and dizzy after passing a black coloured stool in the early hours of the morning. In the ED his pulse rate is 122bpm, BP 100/72mmHg, and respiratory rate 24breaths/min. He is pale, sweaty and anxious. Which is the *single* most appropriate immediate management? ★

A Fresh frozen plasma

B IV proton pump inhibitor

C IV vasopressin

D Normal saline

E O-negative blood

4. A 68-year-old man has had chest pain for the last 5h. He is sweaty and unwell. His pulse is 120bpm, BP 140/90mmHg and respiratory rate 26breaths/min. The ECG is shown in Fig. 3.3. (See the ECG suite at the back of the book for a larger version of this figure →p401.)

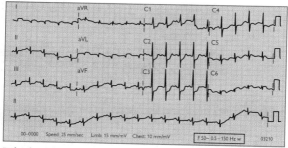

Which is the *single* most likely coronary artery involved? ★

A Circumflex

B Left anterior descending

C Posterior descending

D Right

E Septal

5. A 55-year-old man has had chest pain for the last few hours. He feels nauseous and unwell. His BP is 135/85mmHg and respiratory rate 20breaths/min. The ECG is shown in Fig. 3.4. (See the ECG suite at the back of the book for a larger version of this figure →p402.)

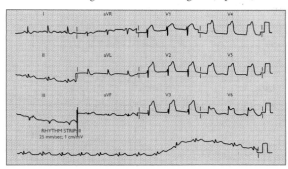

Which is the *single* most appropriate emergency management? ★

A CABG

B Facilitated primary PCI

C Glycoprotein IIb/IIIa receptor inhibitors

D Primary PCI

E Thrombolysis

6. A 58-year-old man has had chest pain for the last 13h. He feels nauseous and unwell. His heart rate is 90bpm, BP 135/85mmHg and respiratory rate 20breaths/min. The ECG is normal. The bloods have been sent to laboratory for analysis. Which is the *single* most specific cardiac marker that may be elevated? ★

A AST

B CK-MB (cardiac isoenzyme)

C LDH

D Myoglobin

E Troponins

7. A 28-year-old man with asthma has been coughing for the past couple of days. He has developed shortness of breath in the past few hours and is finding it difficult to talk. His regular inhalers have not helped him. His PEFR reading is 200L although his usual PEFR is 450L. His heart rate is 112bpm and respiratory rate 30breaths/min. Which is the *single* most appropriate severity of asthma that applies to him? ★

A Acute severe

B Brittle

C Life-threatening

D Moderate exacerbation

E Near fatal

8. A 20-year-old man has suddenly become short of breath with wheezing and now is finding it very difficult to talk. He is asthmatic and his usual inhalers have not helped him. His PEFR is 210L/min and his usual PEFR is 470L/min. He has a temperature 36.8°C, heart rate of 116bpm, respiratory rate of 33breaths/min, and the SaO$_2$ 99% on oxygen. He has been given nebulized β$_2$ agonist and oral prednisolone. He is concerned about taking steroids and asks how they work. What is the *single* most appropriate mechanism of action by which the drug will help in relieving his symptoms? ★

A Bronchial smooth muscle relaxation

B Increased ventilatory drive

C Inhibition of inflammation

D Mechanism unknown

E Mucociliary clearance

9. A 65-year-old fit and healthy man attends the ED with a cough and yellowish sputum that he had had for the last 4 days. His temperature is 38°C, heart rate 116bpm, and respiratory rate 29breaths/min. His chest X-ray is shown in Fig. 3.5.

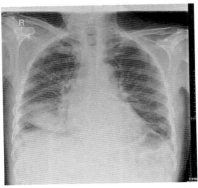

Which is the *single* most likely causative organism? ★

A *Haemophilus influenzae*

B *Legionella pneumophila*

C *Mycoplasma pneumoniae*

D *Staphylococcus aureus*

E *Streptococcus pneumoniae*

10. A 59-year-old man felt dizzy after passing a dark stool. He was treated for a sprain in his right ankle 24h earlier. His pulse rate is 118bpm, BP 100/72mmHg, and respiratory rate 28breaths/min. Which is the *single* most likely cause? ★

A Gastritis

B Mallory–Weiss tear

C Oesophageal varices

D Oesophagitis

E Peptic ulcer

11. A 62-year-old otherwise healthy woman has attended the ED after passing blood and slimy fluid mixed with her stools three times in the last few hours. She has a mild ache in her abdomen. Her temperature is 37°C, pulse rate 102bpm, BP 110/82mmHg, and respiratory rate 20breaths/min. She is tender in the lower abdomen. Which is the *single* most likely cause of the bleeding? ★

A Angiodysplasia

B Colonic malignancy

C Crohn's disease

D Diverticular disease

E Ischaemic colitis

12. A 22-year-old man has had breathlessness, sweating, and vomiting for the last 6h. He has type 1 diabetes. His temperature is 37.8°C, heart rate 120bpm, BP 110/70mmHg, and respiratory rate 34breaths/min. He is alert, does not have any neurological deficit and his capillary blood glucose is 17.8mmol/L. He has been given oxygen 10L/min. The urine dip test shows white cells +, red cells −, ketones +++, glucose +++, and specific gravity 1020. What is the *single* most appropriate emergency fluid management? ★

A 1L colloid over first 30min

B 1L dextrose saline over first 30min

C 1L normal saline over first 30min

D 1L normal saline + potassium 40mmol over first 30min

E 1L normal saline + potassium 40mmol over first 4h

13. A 58-year-old woman attends the ED after feeling unwell and pain around her lower neck for the last 24h. She is under treatment for breast carcinoma with chemotherapy via a Hickman line. Her temperature is 37.7°C, heart rate is 80bpm, BP 120/80mmHg, and respiratory rate 20breaths/min. The Hickman line site looks normal. The WBC count is 1.0×10^9/L. Which is the *single* most appropriate management? ★

A Admitting under the medical team

B Arranging to change the Hickman line

C Discharging her after arranging follow-up with specialist

D Discharging her after reassurance

E Discharging her with oral antibiotics

14. A 52-year-old man has been feeling unwell, lethargic, and weak for the past 2 days. He has type 1 diabetes. His temperature is 37.3°C, heart rate 80bpm, BP 165/100mmHg, and respiratory rate 25breaths/min. His blood results are:

```
sodium 142mmol/L; potassium 6.9mmol/L; urea
12mmol/L; creatinine 600µmol/L; calcium
2.6mmol/L; Hb 12.0g/dL.
```

Which is the *single* most specific treatment? ★

A Calcium chloride IV

B Crystalloid IV

C Diuretics

D Potassium exchange resin

E Sodium bicarbonate

15. ...-year-old previously healthy man has had a ...gh and shortness of breath for the past couple of ... temperature is 37.4°C, heart rate 100bpm, ... mmHg, respiratory rate 24breaths/min, ... on air. His arterial blood gas on air shows:

.49, pCO₂ 3.1 kPa, pO₂ 12.1 kPa, HCO₃– ...mmol/L, BE –0.4mmol/L, and SaO₂ 98%.

... is the *single* most avoidable error that might have ...d the above arterial blood gas reading? ★

A Accidental sampling from vein

B Delayed analysis of the sample

C Exposure to air

D Not using ice while transporting the sample to a nearby machine

E Using at least 1mL of heparin

16. A 30-year-old man has been brought to the ED after being involved in a road traffic incident. He has lost a significant amount of blood from his leg for which he is receiving a blood transfusion. A few minutes later he starts feeling hot and uncomfortable with a rapidly developing itchy rash all over his body. Which is the *single* most appropriate step to take? ★

A Continue transfusion and give hydrocortisone

B Continue transfusion and give paracetamol

C Stop transfusion and give adrenaline (epinephrine)

D Stop transfusion and give chlorphenamine

E Stop transfusion and send the blood bag to the laboratory

17. A 22-year-old man is receiving a blood transfusion in the ED for significant blood following a fall from a scaffolding about 10m high which he sustained a pelvic injury. Five minutes into transfusion he develops a burning sensation at the site infusion, headache, nausea, chills, fever, and chest tightness. Which is the *single* most appropriate important step that could have avoided this? ★

A Accurate labelling of tubes and forms while requesting blood

B Commencing transfusion only by a senior sister

C Giving an antihistamine before starting the transfusion

D Giving blood through the central line

E Taking a history of previous allergic reactions

18. A 66-year-old man with COPD has had a cough and worsening shortness of breath since 5 days. He is bringing up yellowish phlegm with a tinge of red blood. His temperature is 38.0°C, heart rate 112bpm, BP 126/80mmHg, respiratory rate 42breaths/min, and saturation of 88% on air. He has crepitations in the right upper chest with widespread rhonchi and wheeze. His arterial blood gas result on air is:

pH 7.313; pCO_2 7.05kPa; pO_2 6.02kPa; HCO_3^- std 28.6mmol/L; BE -4.07mmol/L

Which is the *single* most appropriate method of initial oxygen therapy? ★

A CPAP

B Hudson mask

C Nasal cannulae

D Reservoir bag

E Venturi mask

19. A 67-year-old previously healthy man has had central chest pain radiating to his left arm for the last 2h. He has type 2 diabetes, hypertension, and has been smoking 10–20 cigarettes per day since the age of 16 years. His heart rate is 100bpm, BP 155/90mmHg and respiratory rate 25breaths/min. The ECG is normal. His troponin level is <0.1μg/L. Which is the *single* most appropriate risk of developing a serious cardiac event within 14 days according to his TIMI score? ★ ★

A 8%

B 13%

C 20%

D 26%

E 41%

20. A 55-year-old man who has been coughing for 3 days is now short of breath. His temperature is 38.5°C, heart rate 110bpm, BP 130/70mmHg, and respiratory rate 35breaths/min. He is conversing normally. His WBC count is 14×10⁹/L, CRP 135mg/L, urea 6.5mmol/L, creatinine 102μmol/L. His chest X-ray shows consolidation in the right mid zone. Which is the *single* most appropriate CURB-65 score? ★ ★

A 1

B 2

C 3

D 4

E 5

21. A 50-year-old previously healthy woman who has been coughing for 3 days is now short of breath. She is wearing nail polish. Her temperature is 38.0°C, heart rate 120bpm, BP 100/75mmHg, respiratory rate 28breaths/min, and SaO$_2$ 88% on air. Her arterial blood gas on air shows:

pH 7.37, pCO$_2$ 4.5kPa, pO$_2$ is 11.1kPa, HCO$_3^-$std 22mmol/L, BE −0.1mmol/L.

Her haemoglobin is 10g/dL and WBC count 11.5×10^9/L. Which is the *single* most likely reason of her reduced SaO$_2$? ★ ★

A Blood pressure

B Chest infection

C Haemoglobin

D Nail polish

E Temperature

22. A 72-year-old man with COPD has sudden right-sided chest pain with shortness of breath. The pain is sharp and gets worse on deep breathing. He has diminished air entry to the right chest with bilateral widespread rhonchi. His respiratory rate is 36 breaths/min with SaO_2 of 93% on air. His chest X-ray is shown in Fig. 3.6.

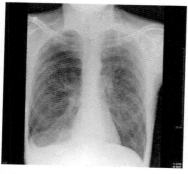

Which is the *single* most appropriate management? ★ ★

A Discharging him with follow-up in chest clinic

B Intercostal tube drainage

C Needle aspiration followed by discharge if successful

D No intervention with advice to return next day for repeat chest X-ray

E No intervention with advice to return only if symptoms get worse

23. A 79-year-old man who has been having increasing shortness of breath and a cough with yellow sputum for 1 week is suddenly experiencing more severe shortness of breath. He has had COPD for 30 years. His heart rate is 100bpm, BP 160/95mmHg, respiratory rate 42breaths/min, and SaO_2 86% on air. Chest examination reveals widespread bilateral wheeze, rhonchi, and crepitations. Which is the *single* most likely arterial blood gas result? ★ ★

A pH 7.163; pCO_2 4.05kPa; pO_2 15.0kPa; HCO_3^- std 15.6mmol/L; BE −9.87mmol/L; FiO_2 100%

B pH 7.255; pCO_2 8.81kPa; pO_2 6.35kPa; HCO_3^- std 28.7mmol/L; BE −0.3mmol/L; FiO_2 28%

C pH 7.355; pCO_2 4.51kPa; pO_2 9.35kPa; HCO_3^- std 20.2mmol/L; BE −0.1mmol/L; FiO_2 air

D pH 7.355; pCO_2 4.05kPa; pO_2 6.25kPa; HCO_3^- std 25.6mmol/L; BE −0.1mmol/L; FiO_2 air

E pH 7.555; pCO_2 3.07kPa; pO_2 12.51kPa; HCO_3^- std 21.4mmol/L; BE −1.1mmol/L; FiO_2 air

24. A 72-year-old man who has had a cough and fever for the last week has now suddenly become short of breath and coughed up a cup full of fresh blood. His temperature is 38.6°C, heart rate 126bpm, BP 150/85mmHg, respiratory rate 43breaths/min, and SaO_2 98% on 10 L/min of oxygen. IV cannulation is done. Which is the *single* most appropriate next step in the initial management? ★ ★

A Antibiotics

B Arterial blood gas

C Blood culture

D Chest X-ray

E ECG

25. A 68-year-old man with a hiatus hernia collapsed and fainted for a brief period after vomiting a large amount of dark and fresh blood. His pulse rate is 124bpm, BP 96/70mmHg, and respiratory rate 24 breaths/min. On admission he is pale, sweaty, and anxious. Which is the *single* most severe class of haemorrhage? ★ ★

A Class I

B Class II

C Class III

D Class IV

E Class V

26. A 72-year-old man developed sudden-onset, right-sided weakness of the face, arm, and leg, and difficulty talking 2h ago. On his arrival in the ED, he has recovered completely. His heart rate is 72bpm, BP 165/95mmHg, and respiratory rate 18breaths/min. He is alert and has a normal neurological examination. What is his risk of developing a stroke within the next 48h? ★ ★

A 0%

B 1%

C 4%

D 5%

E 8%

27. A 32-year-old man who is on long-term treatment for seizures has had a generalized convulsion after being fit-free for 2 years. The seizure stopped before his arrival in the ED. He has been on carbamazepine 1g daily for many years. He had 5 pints of lager at a party yesterday. He is now alert and has no neurological deficits. His routine blood test results are normal. Which is the *single* most appropriate management? ★ ★

A Admitting under medical team for 24h neuro-observation

B Arranging a CT scan of the brain

C Discharging him after increasing the dose of carbamazepine

D Discharging him with advice to avoid alcohol

E Referral to neurology outpatients

28. A 22-year-old previously healthy man has had a sudden generalized convulsion which stopped before his arrival at the ED. His temperature is 38.2°C, heart rate 90bpm, BP 120/70mmHg, and respiratory rate 20breaths/min. He is now alert and does not have any neurological deficits. The bedside glucose is 4.8mmol/L. Which is the *single* most appropriate initial management? ★ ★

A Admitting under the medical team for observation

B Arranging a CT scan of the brain

C Discharging him after starting antiepileptic medication

D Discharging him with advice to see his GP

E Referral to neurology outpatients

29. A 32-year-old man with sickle cell disease has been having severe pain in his upper abdomen for the last couple of hours. He is now writhing in pain and asking for morphine. He has been admitted with similar symptoms several times in the past. His temperature is 37.4°C, heart rate 90bpm, BP 112/80mmHg, respiratory rate 24breaths/min, and SaO₂ 97% on air. Which is the *single* most appropriate step to take? ★ ★

A Confirming sickling on blood film before giving him morphine

B Confirming sickling by testing for blood in a urine dipstick before giving him analgesia

C Discharging him after giving NSAIDs as he is probably a morphine addict

D Giving morphine IV as he requests

E Withholding morphine until splenomegaly is confirmed

30. A 27-year-old man has had a stabbing pain in the centre of his chest for the past 2 days. The pain radiates to his left arm and upper abdomen, and worsens on lying flat and deep breathing. He has smoked 20 cigarettes/day since the age of 14. His heart rate is 108bpm, BP 125/85mmHg and respiratory rate 23breaths/min. The ECG is shown in Fig. 3.7.

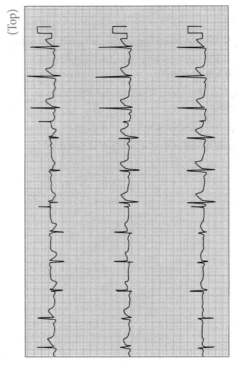

(Top)

Which is the *single* most appropriate emergency treatment? ★ ★ ★

A Antiplatelet agent

B NSAIDs

C Pericardiocentesis

D Primary PCI

E Thrombolytic agent

31. A 60-year-old man has had chest pain for the last 4h. He is on atenolol 50mg a day for hypertension. His BP is 170/110mmHg and respiratory rate 20breaths/min. His chest is clear. The serum urea is 10mmol/L and creatinine 191μmol/L. The ECG is shown in Fig. 3.8.

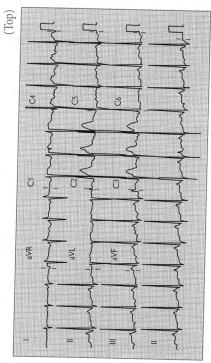

Which is the *single* most appropriate treatment? ★ ★ ★

A Arranging monitoring and follow-up by GP

B Discharging him after increasing the dose of atenolol and outpatient follow-up

C Discharging him after reassurance and dietary advice

D Referral to the medical team for admission and treatment

E Starting an additional antihypertensive agent and arrange follow-up by GP

32. A 62-year-old man has had a headache for the past 6h and has been sick three times. He is on atenolol 50mg a day for hypertension. He is alert and orientated. His heart rate is 64bpm, BP 190/130mmHg, and respiratory rate 22breaths/min. His chest is clear. The serum urea is 12mmol/L and creatinine is 191μmol/L. Which is the *single* most appropriate management? ★ ★ ★

A Giving additional antihypertensive orally and admitting under the medical team

B Giving analgesics and changing the antihypertensive agent

C Increasing the regular dose of atenolol and arranging urgent follow-up with GP

D IV antihypertensive agent given urgently and admitting to hospital

E Starting additional antihypertensive agent and follow-up with GP

33. A 55-year-old healthy man has vomited yellowish fluid a number of times last night after drinking 8 pints of lager. He has also been retching and has noted a streak of fresh blood on a couple of recent occasions of vomiting. His temperature is 37°C, pulse rate 90bpm, BP 130/85mmHg, and respiratory rate 20breaths/min. Which is the *single* most appropriate way to stop the bleeding? ★ ★ ★

A Embolization by selective arteriography

B Endoscopic cauterization

C No active measure required

D Surgical over-sewing of bleeding points

E Tamponade with a Sengstaken–Blakemore tube

34. A 75-year-old man developed sudden-onset left-sided weakness of his face, arm and leg about an hour ago. He also has reduced sensation in these areas. He is alert and has ipsilateral hemianopia. He is unable to move the left upper limb, but he can move the left leg from side to side. Jerks are absent in the upper limbs but are weakly present in the lower limbs. The patient is unable close his eyelids, puff out his cheeks or whistle, and exposes his teeth on the right when asked to smile. Which is the *single* most likely arterial territory involved? ★ ★ ★

A Anterior cerebral

B Lacunar

C Middle cerebral

D Posterior cerebral

E Vertebral

35. A 68-year-old man has been brought in by a blue light ambulance as he was found lying on the floor in his flat by his son. He has COPD, and is on home oxygen therapy with nebulizers and steroids. His temperature is 35.1°C, heart rate 110bpm, BP 78/50mmHg, respiratory rate 28breaths/min, and SaO_2 91%. His capillary blood glucose is 4.0mmol/L and GCS score 12/15 (E3, M5, V4). He has multiple bruises on his limbs and body. His arterial blood gases are as follows:

pH 7.313; pCO_2 5.82kPa; pO_2 9.02kPa; HCO_3^- std 28.6mmol/L; BE −5.07mmol/L; FiO_2 31%.

Which is the *single* most appropriate emergency management? ★ ★ ★ ★

A Antibiotics IV

B Glucose IV

C Hydrocortisone IV

D Increase FiO_2 to 35%

E Sodium bicarbonate IV

$36.$ A 61-year-old woman who is a social drinker has had diarrhoea and vomiting for the past 5 days. She is now apathetic and anorexic, with confusion developing over the last couple of days. She has Addison's disease and is on steroids. Her temperature is 35.5°C, heart rate 110bpm, BP 95/70mmHg, and respiratory rate 24breaths/min. The capillary blood glucose is 5.8mmol/L. She has been given oxygen 10L/min.

Which is the *single* most likely underlying cause of her recent deterioration?★ ★ ★ ★

A Alcohol consumption

B Dehydration

C Hypothermia

D Infection

E Sudden withdrawal of steroid therapy

37. A 28-year-old man with sickle cell disease has had severe pain in his right chest, a cough and shortness of breath in the last couple of hours. His temperature is 38.1°C, heart rate 110bpm, BP 110/75mmHg, respiratory rate 34breaths/min, and SaO_2 90% on air. His chest X-ray is shown in Fig. 3.9.

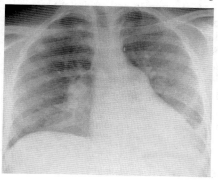

Which is the *single* most likely diagnosis? ★ ★ ★ ★

A Acute chest syndrome

B Adult respiratory distress syndrome

C Congestive heart failure

D Pneumonia

E Pulmonary embolism

38. A 72-year-old man has been feeling lethargic and nauseous, and has had pain in the abdomen for the last week. His symptoms are gradually worsening. He has not opened his bowels for about 5 days, which is unusual for him. He was treated for squamous carcinoma of the lung 3 weeks ago. His temperature is 36.9°C, heart rate 60bpm, BP 165/100mmHg, and respiratory rate 22breaths/min. His haemoglobin is 10g/dL, WBC count is 4.0×10^9/L, sodium 142mmol/L, potassium 4.5mmol/L, calcium (corrected) 3.1mmol/L, urea 7.5mmol/L, and creatinine 176µmol/L. He has been given oxygen. Which is the *single* most appropriate management? ★ ★ ★ ★

A 0.9% normal saline

B Calcitonin

C Dialysis

D Glucocorticoid

E Sodium pamidronate

39. An 89-year-old man attends the ED for severe back pain experienced in the past few hours. He has terminal metastatic prostatic carcinoma with secondaries in the spine. He has recently signed an advance directive for 'do-not-attempt-resuscitation' in the event of cardiac arrest. His heart rate is 60bpm, BP 110/80mmHg, and respiratory rate 14breaths/min. He has been given oxygen. Which is the *single* most appropriate immediate management? ★ ★ ★ ★

A Admit under Orthopaedics team for further investigation

B Arranging imaging of the spine

C 'Do not attempt resuscitation' as stated in the advance directive

D Giving appropriate analgesics to make him comfortable

E Referral to an anaesthetist for spinal injection

40. A 22-year-old woman who has longstanding asthma, has been experiencing shortness of breath for the past few hours. She has been also coughing for the last 2 days and her usual inhalers have not helped her. Her PEFR is 230L and her usual PEFR is 450L. Her heart rate is 110bpm, respiratory rate 30breaths/min, and SaO_2 94% on air. After treating her with nebulized bronchodilators and steroids, her PEFR is 350L/min, respiratory rate 26breaths/min, heart rate 110bpm, and SaO2 96%. Which is the *single* most appropriate next management? ★ ★ ★ ★

A Admitting to hospital for further nebulizer treatment

B Discharging her with antibiotics

C Discharging her with follow-up by GP

D Discharging her with follow-up in outpatients

E Discharging her with no follow-up

Medicine

EXTENDED MATCHING QUESTIONS

Clinical diagnosis of chest pain

For each of the following scenarios, choose the clinical features and/or observations from the list of options below to clinch the most likely diagnosis. Each option may be used once, more than once, or not at all.

A Absent left femoral pulse

B Absent right femoral pulse

C Bilateral crepitations and wheeze

D Early diastolic murmur at the left sternal edge

E Ejection systolic murmur with radiation to neck

F Finger clubbing

G Focal crepitations and bronchial breathing

H Mid-diastolic murmur

I Pansystolic murmur at the apex radiating to the axilla

J Percussion of the chest

K Raised jugular venous pulsation and bilateral crepitations in the chest.

L Systolic and diastolic creaking sound heard over the left sternal edge

M Tender and swollen calf

N Tender and swollen costal cartilages

1. A 45-year-old previously healthy man has had a central, sharp chest pain for the past 12h, which started gradually and is now getting worse. The pain is worse on coughing, inspiration, and arm movements. His heart rate is 90bpm, BP 132/85mmHg, respiratory rate 22 breaths/min, and temperature 37.3°C. His heart sounds and ECG are normal.

2. A 35-year man has had stabbing central chest pain for the last 10h. The pain started gradually and worsens when he lies down or coughs. His heart rate is 100bpm, BP 140/80mmHg, respiratory rate 22 breaths/min, and temperature 37°C. The ECG is normal.

3. An 82-year-old man had sudden onset of severe, central chest pain 1h ago. He felt the pain in his back as well and passed out for a brief period. He has been on atenolol for hypertension for many years. His heart rate is 110bpm, BP 100/70mmHg, and respiratory rate 28 breaths/min. He has a soft second heart sound.

4. A 58-year-old man had sudden onset of severe chest pain and shortness of breath 3h ago. The pain is radiating to his left arm, and he is unwell and sweaty. His heart rate is 120bpm, BP 100/90mmHg, respiratory rate 26 breaths/min, and SaO$_2$ 90%. The ECG is normal.

5. A 37-year-old woman has had sudden onset of right-sided sharp chest pain and shortness of breath. She has recently been treated conservatively for a fracture of her left ankle. Her heart rate is 130bpm, BP 100/85mmHg, respiratory rate 38 breaths/min, temperature 37.2°C, and SaO$_2$ 90% on air. There is bilateral equal air entry with no added sounds. The ECG shows sinus tachycardia.

Emergency management of arrhythmias

For each of the following scenarios, choose the most appropriate emergency management from the list of options below. Each option may be used once, more than once, or not at all.

A Adenosine

B Amiodarone

C Atropine

D Digoxin

E Esmolol

F Flecainide

G Magnesium sulphate

H No emergency treatment required

I Shock

J Synchronized DC shock

K Verapamil

6. A 65-year-old man has had central chest discomfort, shortness of breath, and palpitations during the last 12h; the symptoms developed gradually but are now getting worse. His BP is 95/65mmHg and respiratory rate 32 breaths/min. There are bilateral crepitations in the chest with pedal pitting oedema. The ECG is shown in Fig. 3.10.

(Top)

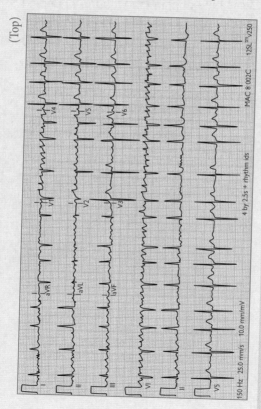

(See the ECG suite at the back of the book for larger versions
of Figures 3.11 →p403 and 3.12 →p404 in this EMQ.)

7. A 35-year-old man has had sudden onset of
palpitations 2h ago. In the ED, his BP is
110/80mmHg and respiratory rate 20 breaths/min.
The ECG is shown in Fig. 3.11.

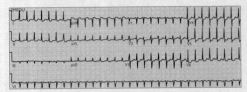

8. A 72-year-old man has had fatigue and shortness
of breath while walking to the newsagent in the past
3 days. He also suddenly feels dizzy when climbing
stairs rapidly. His BP is 90/64mmHg and respiratory
rate 24 breaths/min. His cardiovascular examination
is normal and the ECG is shown in Fig. 3.12.

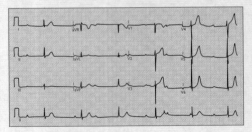

9. A 62-year-old man developed sudden-onset
shortness of breath and palpitations 3h ago. He had
an acute myocardial infarction 5 years ago. His BP is
150/90mmHg and respiratory rate 26 breaths/min.
The ECG is shown in Fig. 3.13.

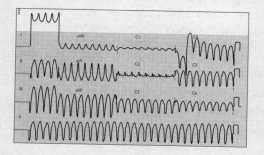

10. A 21-year-old previously healthy woman has had sudden onset of dizziness and palpitations an hour ago; these have now settled and she is feeling fine. Her BP is 120/75mmHg, respiratory rate 22 breaths/min, and SaO$_2$ 98% on air. Clinical examination is normal. The rhythm strip is shown in Fig. 3.14.

(Top)

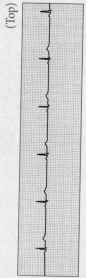

Clinical diagnosis of breathlessness

For each of the following scenarios, choose the additional clinical features and/or observations which may be present, from the list of options below, to clinch the most likely diagnosis. Each option may be used once, more than once, or not at all.

A Bilateral crepitations and wheeze
B Bilateral hyperresonance on chest percussion
C Bilateral polyphonic diffuse expiratory wheeze
D Bronchial breath sounds
E Dullness on contralateral chest percussion
F Dullness on ipsilateral chest percussion
G Finger clubbing
H Focal crepitations and bronchial breathing
I Hyperresonant on contralateral chest percussion
J Hyperresonant on ipsilateral chest percussion
K Stony dullness on percussion

11. A 25-year-old healthy man is experiencing sudden-onset shortness of breath and sharp chest pain on the right side. His heart rate is 90bpm, BP 112/75mmHg, respiratory rate 32 breaths/min, and SaO$_2$ 90% on air. The right-sided chest movement and air entry are reduced. The heart sounds are normal.

12. A 20-year-old asthmatic woman has had a cough with chest tightness for the past 2 days, which are worse in the early morning. She has suddenly become short of breath in the last couple of hours and is unable to talk. Her heart rate is 120bpm, BP 110/80mmHg, respiratory rate 42 breaths/min, and SaO$_2$ 88% on air. There are equal bilateral chest movements and air entry.

13. A 42-year-old man has had a cough with yellowish-green expectoration for the past 3 days. He has suddenly become short of breath in the past few hours. His heart rate is 130bpm, BP 120/80mmHg, respiratory rate 38 breaths/min, temperature 38.3°C, and SaO$_2$ 90% on air. There is diminished air entry with local fine crackles, dullness on percussion, and increased vocal resonance in the left lower base.

14. A 58-year-old man who has been short of breath for the past few weeks has become suddenly worse in the past 3h. He has had chest pain on the right side for the past couple of days. He is unwell and sweaty. His heart rate is 130bpm, BP 100/90mmHg, respiratory rate 38 breaths/min, temperature 38°C, and SaO$_2$ is 94%. Air entry and vocal resonance is diminished in the right lower chest.

15. A 69-year-old man has had increasing shortness of breath and an early morning cough for 1 week. He has been smoking 40 cigarettes/day for the past 42 years. His heart rate is 90bpm, BP 160/95mmHg, respiratory rate 38 breaths/min, and SaO_2 90% on air. The chest has bilaterally reduced movement with quiet breath sounds and hyperinflation.

Clinical/radiological diagnosis of breathlessness/cough

For each of the following scenarios, choose the most likely clinical or radiological diagnosis from the list of options below. Each option may be used once, more than once, or not at all.

A Cavitations

B Collapse

C Consolidation

D Malignancy

E Normal

F Pleural effusion

G Pneumothorax

H Pulmonary oedema

I Tension pneumothorax

16. A 20-year-old healthy man has sudden-onset shortness of breath. Right-sided chest movement and air entry is reduced. His chest X-ray is shown in Fig. 3.15.

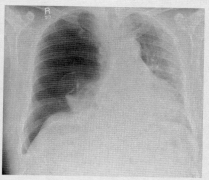

17. A 58-year-old man has been having shortness of breath for the past few weeks, which suddenly worsened 3h ago. He also has had chest pain on the right side for the past 2 days. His chest X-ray is shown in Fig. 3.16.

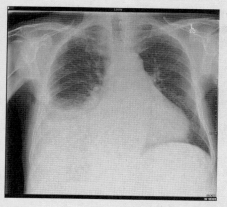

18. A 72-year-old woman has had a cough with yellowish-green expectoration for 1 week. She suddenly became short of breath a few hours ago and has coughed up a cupful of fresh blood. Her chest X-ray is shown in Fig. 3.17.

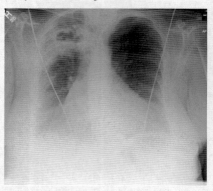

19. A 78-year-old woman who has been short of breath and has had a cough for the past few weeks has become suddenly worse in the past 3h. She had an acute myocardial infarction 5 years ago. She is unwell and sweaty. Her chest X-ray is shown in Fig. 3.18.

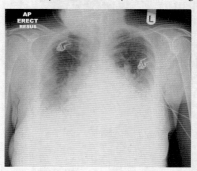

20. A 65-year-old woman has had a fever, cough with yellow sputum, and shortness of breath for the past 4 days. Her heart rate is 110bpm, BP 160/95mmHg, respiratory rate 38 breaths/min, temperature 38.9°C, and SaO$_2$ 90% on air. Her chest X-ray is shown in Fig. 3.19.

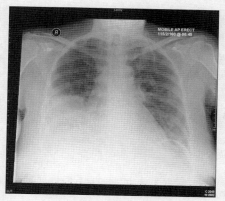

Aetiology of acute diarrhoea

For each of the following scenarios, choose the most likely causative organism from the list of options below. Each option may be used once, more than once, or not at all.

A *Bacillus cereus*

B *Campylobacter* spp.

C *Clostridium difficile*

D *Escherichia coli*

E *Entamoeba histolytica*

F *Giardia*

G *Norovirus*

H *Rotavirus*

I *Salmonella* spp.

J *Shigella*

K *Staphylococcus* spp.

L *Vibrio cholerae*

21. A 25-year-old healthcare worker in a nursing home has passed watery stools without blood 10–12 times and has vomited three times within the past 12h. He has also felt unwell and feverish for the past 2 days. His heart rate is 90bpm, BP is 112/75mmHg, respiratory rate 18 breaths/min, and temperature 37.5°C. His central abdomen is mildly tender but there is no rebound or guarding.

22. A 30-year-old woman has had abdominal pain, fever, and a headache for the past 24h. She now has passed watery stools with blood six to eight times in the past 12h. She ate left-over chicken about 24h earlier. Her temperature is 39°C, heart rate 120bpm, BP 110/80mmHg, and respiratory rate 18 breaths/min. Her abdomen is soft but tender in the lower part on both sides.

23. An 85-year-old woman has been transferred from a nursing home after having six episodes of large watery stools without blood but associated with lower abdominal cramps for 1 day. She has type 2 diabetes and a UTI was treated with a course of quinolones 3 weeks ago. Her temperature is 37°C, heart rate 90bpm, BP 150/90mmHg, and respiratory rate 18 breaths/min. Her abdomen is diffusely, mildly tender, mostly in the left lower part.

24. A 28-year-old man has had an abrupt onset of watery diarrhoea with no blood, with six to eight episodes over the past 12h. He returned from a trekking holiday in Bolivia 2 days ago. His temperature is 37.1°C, heart rate 70bpm, BP 118/72mmHg, and respiratory rate 16 breaths/min. He has associated mild abdominal cramps. He does not feel unwell.

25. A 32-year-old woman has had a sudden onset of bouts of crampy abdominal pain, violent vomiting and a couple of episodes of mild watery stool without blood in the past few hours after having a takeaway meal. Her temperature is 36.8°C, heart rate 82bpm, BP 130/80mmHg, and respiratory rate 20 breaths/min. She is otherwise well.

Cause of syncope

For each of the following scenarios, choose the most likely diagnosis from the list of options below. Each option may be used once, more than once, or not at all.

A AAA rupture

B Aortic dissection

C Cardiac tamponade

D Critical aortic stenosis

E Hypertrophic cardiomyopathy

F Life-threatening dysrhythmias

G Myocardial infarction

H Pulmonary embolism

I Severe hypovolaemia

J Stroke

K Subarachnoid haemorrhage

L Subdural haemorrhage

M Upper GI haemorrhage

N Vasovagal syncope

26. A 45-year-old previously healthy man is brought to the ED after suddenly passing out for a brief period while digging in the garden. His heart rate is 80bpm, BP 110/60mmHg, and respiratory rate 28 breaths/min. He is short of breath and has a systolic murmur in the precordial area with radiation to the neck. The ECG shows a tall R wave in aV_L and I, V_{4-6}, deep S wave in V_1, and widespread ST depression and T wave inversion.

27. A 75-year-old man has severe, sharp central chest and back pain, which started suddenly 1h ago. He passed out for a brief period. The pain has eased off now, but he is short of breath. He has been under treatment for hypertension for many years. His heart rate is 100bpm, BP 90/60mmHg, and respiratory rate 24 breaths/min. He has a short, soft diastolic murmur in the precordium. The ECG is normal.

28. A 72-year-old man with sudden onset of right-sided chest pain passed out for a brief period. On regaining consciousness he is short of breath and feeling unwell. He was treated for prostatic carcinoma by radiotherapy followed by surgery 6 weeks earlier. His heart rate is 110bpm, BP 100/70mmHg, and respiratory rate 38 breaths/min. The ECG shows tachycardia and the SaO_2 is 90% on high-flow oxygen.

29. A 68-year-old man drives to the ED after having a fainting episode with sudden onset of severe abdominal and low back pain. His heart rate is 80bpm, BP 110/80mmHg and respiratory rate 24 breaths/min. His heart examination is normal but he has minimal tenderness in the epigastrium. The ECG is normal.

30. A 57-year-old previously healthy man attends the ED after collapsing on a sofa while feeling dizzy and having moderate chest pain. The pain is slightly worse now and feels like an ache across the front of his chest. He is slightly short of breath. His heart rate is 90bpm, respiratory rate 24 breaths/min and BP 140/95mmHg. The ECG shows tall R waves in V_{1-2}, ST depression in V_{1-3}, tall and wide T waves, ST elevation on V_{4-6}, I, and aV_L.

Diagnosis of headache

For each of the following scenarios, choose the most likely diagnosis from the list of options below.
Each option may be used once, more than once, or not at all.

A Benign cough headache

B Benign intracranial hypertension

C Brain tumour

D Cluster headache

E Depression

F Giant cell arteritis

G Intracranial hypertension

H Meningitis

I Migraine

J Stroke

K Subarachnoid haemorrhage

L Subdural haemorrhage

M Tension headache

31. A 25-year-old woman has had generalized headaches for the past 5 days. The pain started with low intensity, as a dull ache in the occipital area then becoming generalized. The intensity has remained the same. She does not have any associated nausea or vomiting. She has never had any headaches in the past. Examination is normal except some tenderness around the scalp.

32. A 42-year-old woman had a sudden-onset, severe, generalized headache while watching television the previous night. She felt nauseous and dizzy at the time of onset, and vomited once. The pain lasted for about half an hour before becoming a persistent dull ache. She has never had a headache in the past. Physical examination is normal.

33. A 72-year-old woman has had a throbbing headache for the past 6–8h. It started gradually on the left side but is now getting worse and becoming generalized. There is no associated nausea or vomiting. She has had headaches in the past but this episode is different. She has tenderness on the sides of the scalp but the rest of the examination is normal.

34. A 68-year-old man with type 2 diabetes has had a right-sided headache for 12h. It started gradually but is now throbbing and severe. He has vomited a few times, and he feels unwell and feverish. He is avoiding light and is becoming irritable. He has a temperature of 38.5°C, heart rate of 110bpm, and BP 140/85mmHg. He has difficulty in moving his neck.

35. A 77-year-old previously healthy man attends the ED with a generalized headache that he has experienced for the past 3 weeks; the headache began after he was mugged and is temporarily relieved by analgesics, but it is now getting gradually worse. He has become irritable and prefers to curl up and sleep most of the time. He is avoiding conversation and light but otherwise his neurological examination is normal.

Emergency management of coma

For each of the following scenarios, choose the most appropriate immediate management from the list of options below. Each option may be used once, more than once, or not at all.

A Airway protection

B Antibiotics IV

C Cervical spine protection

D Crystalloid IV

E CT scan of brain

F Glucose IV

G Lumbar puncture

H Mannitol IV

 I Naloxone IV

J Near-patient testing of capillary blood glucose

K Steroid IV

36. A 45-year-old man has been brought to the ED with sudden collapse and loss of consciousness. An oropharyngeal airway has been inserted and he has been given oxygen at the rate of 10L/min. His heart rate is 100bpm, BP 110/80mmHg, and respiratory rate 18 breaths/min. The pupils are 3mm on each side and reacting sluggishly to light. He has needle marks on his abdomen.

37. A young woman has been found unconscious in a city centre. She does not open her eyes on stimulation and shows no verbal or motor response. Her heart rate is 50bpm, BP 100/70mmHg, respiratory rate 10 breaths/min, and near-patient capillary glucose 5.1mmol/L. Her pupils are 2mm and reacting to light. An anaesthetist has been called for endotracheal intubation. An oropharyngeal airway is been inserted and she is given oxygen at the rate of 15L/min.

38. A 56-year-old woman who has had a headache for the past hour suddenly collapses and becomes unconscious. Her heart rate is 55bpm, BP 156/100mmHg, and respiratory rate 12 breaths/min. She opens her eyes to painful stimulus, makes only sounds and hyperextends the limbs on applying a stimulus. The right pupil is 4mm and left 3mm, and the plantars are upgoing.

39. A 70-year-old man has been found unconscious at home. His heart rate is 120bpm, BP 120/85mmHg, temperature 35.5°C, and respiratory rate 20 breaths/min. He does not open his eyes on stimulation and shows no verbal or motor response. The pupils are 3mm on each side and reacting to light. There are no focal neurological signs. The near-patient capillary glucose is >30mmol/L. His airway has been protected.

40. A 22-year-old previously healthy woman has been found unconscious in the university halls. There is no evidence of any trauma. Her temperature is 38.9°C, heart rate 120bpm, BP 90/70mmHg, and respiratory rate 25 breaths/min. She opens her eyes to painful stimulus, making incomprehensible sounds, and shows no motor response. Her neck appears stiff. She has been intubated and given crystalloid. Her near-patient capillary glucose is 5.3mmol/L.

Management of acute heart failure

For each of the following scenarios, choose the most appropriate emergency management from the list of options below. Each option may be used once, more than once, or not at all.

A Anticholinergic agent

B AV node-blocking agent

C β-blocker

D Continuous positive airway pressure therapy

E Fluid challenge

F Loop diuretic

G Non-loop diuretic

H Opioid

 I Oxygen therapy

J Propped-up position

K Synchronized electrical cardioversion

L Vasodilator

41. A 75-year-old man has had a sudden onset of central chest discomfort, palpitations, and shortness of breath in the past 12h. He has been getting increasingly breathless in the past week. He had an acute myocardial infarction 7 years ago and has hypertension and type 2 diabetes. His BP is 152/95mmHg, respiratory rate 32 breaths/min, and SaO_2 88% on air and he has pedal pitting oedema. There are bilateral crepitations in the chest and gallop rhythm. He is in the propped-up position. The ECG is shown in Fig. 3.20.

(Top)

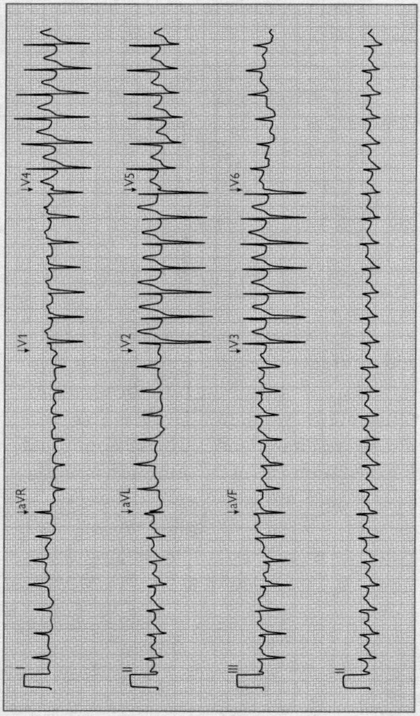

(See the ECG suite at the back of the book for larger
versions of the following figures in this EMQ.)

42. An 85-year-old man has palpitations and
shortness of breath which started suddenly about 3h
ago. He has been coughing for the past couple of
weeks. He has ischaemic heart disease and
hypertension. His BP is 172/100mmHg, respiratory
rate 38 breaths/min, and SaO$_2$ 90% on air. He has
pitting oedema in both feet. On auscultation, there
are crepitations on both sides of the chest and
gallop rhythm in the precordium. The patient is
in the propped-up position and is receiving oxygen
via a non-rebreathing mask. The ECG is shown
in Fig. 3.21→p405.

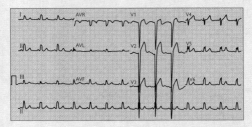

43. A 78-year-old woman has had a gradual onset of
cough and shortness of breath on exertion for the
past 3–4 weeks. She attends the ED with a sudden
exaggeration of her symptoms. Her BP is
130/85mmHg, respiratory rate 30 breaths/min, and
saturation of 98% on 15L of oxygen. She has bilateral,
widespread crepitations and wheeze in the chest.
The heart sounds are soft with gallop rhythm. She is
propped up, and given oxygen, morphine, and
furosemide. The ECG is shown in Fig. 3.22→p406.

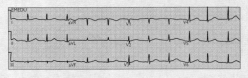

44. A 62-year-old man has had sudden onset of shortness of breath and chest tightness in the past 3h. He has smoked 25–30 cigarettes/day since the age of 16. His BP is 85/60mmHg, respiratory rate 36 breaths/min, and SaO₂ 90% on 15L/min of oxygen. He has scattered bilateral crepitations in the chest and gallop rhythm. He has been propped up and given morphine IV. The ECG is shown in Fig. 3.23 →p407.

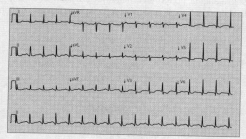

45. A 71-year-old woman has had worsening breathlessness for the past 3h. She has been short of breath for the past couple of weeks. She has ischaemic heart disease, hypertension, and arthritis. She is on a number of medications. Her BP is 120/75mmHg, respiratory rate 42 breaths/min, and SaO₂ 88% on 15L/min of oxygen. She has already received the initial standard treatment without much improvement. The ECG is shown in Fig. 3.24 →p408.

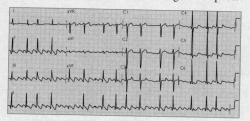

Single Best Answers

1. C ★

ACS (unstable angina, non-ST elevation myocardial infarction, and myocardial infarction) is initiated by endothelial damage and rupture or fissuring of the atheromatous plaque. This in turn results in platelet aggregation and thrombus formation. As a result of the damage, vasospasm is induced by local inflammatory mediators causing further reduction in the blood supply to the myocardium. The ECG in Fig. 3.1 shows ST elevation in V_2, V_3, I, aVL with reciprocal changes in inferior leads (II, III, and aVF).

Advanced Life Support Manual, UK Resuscitation Council.

2. D ★   OHEM, 4th edn → p76

Localization of myocardial infarction: elevation of ST segment more than 1mm in leads II, III, and aVF occurs in inferior acute myocardial infarction. In the chest leads, the elevation of ST segment should be a minimum of 2mm to diagnose acute myocardial infarction.

- Anterior: V_{2-4}
- Anterolateral = V_{5-6}, aV_L
- Anteroseptal = V_{1-3}
- Extensive anterior = V_{1-6}
- Posterior = Reciprocal changes in V_{1-3} and ST elevation in V_{7-9}.

For additional information, see *Emergencies in Clinical Medicine*, p136.

3. D ★   OHEM, 4th edn → pp126–7

Insert two large IV cannulae and start IV fluids immediately.

A: There is no indication for giving fresh frozen plasma.

B: IV proton pump inhibitors are only indicated after endoscopy and once a peptic ulcer is diagnosed to reduce chances of re-bleeding. According to SIGN guidelines, proton pump inhibitors should not be used prior to diagnosis by endoscopy in patients presenting with acute upper gastrointestinal bleeding. One RCT suggested that high-dose omeprazole infusion (80 mg bolus followed by 8 mg/hour) prior to endoscopy accelerated the signs of resolution of bleeding and reduced the need for endoscopic therapy (see the reference below). This study may not be generalizable to Scotland/the UK as it was carried out in an Asian population. The treatment effect is higher in Asian patients who are more sensitive to PPI treatment. The study also excluded patients on long-term aspirin therapy. The optimum dose and route of PPI is unclear and requires to be evaluated in a non-Asian population.

C: IV vasopressin is not indicated.

E: There is no rush to transfuse O-negative blood. A blood sample for proper cross-matching should be taken when inserting the IV cannula. If the patient does not respond to the IV fluids or deteriorates further, a group-specific or crossed-match blood is a safer option than O-negative blood.

Lau JY, Leung WK, Wu JC, Chan FK, Wong VW, Chiu PW, et al. Omeprazole before endoscopy in patients with gastrointestinal bleeding. *N Eng J Med* 2007;356(16):1631-40.

Oxford Handbook of Acute Medicine, 3rd edn, p226.

→ www.sign.ac.uk/pdf/sign105.pdf

4. A ★   OHEM, 4th edn → p76

Localization of myocardial infarction: tall R waves and ST segment depression in V_{1-3} and V_6 are highly suspicious of a posterior myocardial infarction. The diagnosis may be confirmed by performing an ECG after placing the leads on the posterior axillary line (V_7), at the inferior angle of scapula (V_8) and in between the spines and V_8 (V_9).

A: posterior myocardial infarction is caused by blockage in the circumflex coronary artery.

B: Blockage in left anterior descending artery causes anterolateral and anteroseptal myocardial infarction.

C: The posterior descending artery is a branch of right coronary artery supplying the inferior wall of the left ventricle and inferior third of the interventricular septum.

D: The right coronary artery supplies the sinoatrial and AV nodes, and the right ventricle.

E: Septal arteries are branches from the left anterior descending artery and supply the anterior two-thirds of the ventricular septum.

Fig. 3.25 shows the coronary artery anatomy and Table 3.1 shows the coronary artery territories (see *Emergencies in Cardiology*, 2nd edn, pp42–3).

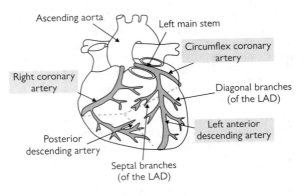

Fig. 3.25

Table 3.1 Coronary artery territories

Site of arterial occlusion	Myocardial territory	ECG changes
LAD	Anterolateral	V_4–V_6, I, VL
	Anteroseptal	V_1–V_4 LBBB
LCX	Posterior	Mirror image changes in V_1–V_2 or V_3, i.e. ST segment depression ± inferior changes; tall R in V1; may be electrically silent on standard 12-lead ECG
RCA	Inferior wall of left ventricle	II, III, aVF
	Right ventricle	ST elevation V_{4R}–V_{6R}

5. D ★

Primary PCI is the treatment of choice and should be performed within 60min of arrival to the department (door-to-balloon time); the purpose is to restore the myocardial perfusion as soon as possible.

A: CABG is not usually done urgently, but may be required if PCI has failed.

B: Facilitated primary PCI is using lytic therapy in full or partial dosage prior to primary PCI, and is not recommended at present because of lack of benefit and increased chances of bleeding.

C: Giving glycoprotein IIb/IIIA prior to primary PCI does not improve long-term outcomes. It is given as bolus and infusion in hours after the primary PCI.

E: Thrombolysis in only reserved for the units where primary PCI is not available as the latter is the preferred treatment.

For additional information, see *Emergencies in Cardiology*, 2nd edn, pp48–54.

6. E ★   OHEM, 4th edn → p73

Troponins are contractile proteins, specific to the myocardium. Their level is elevated in myocardial infarction. It starts rising within 12h, peaking at around 24h. The role of traditional cardiac enzymes is reducing as the troponin is now used universally. However it is important to remember that troponin T may be elevated in myocarditis, pericarditis, pulmonary embolism, sepsis, and renal failure. The test should be done at 12h after onset of pain in order to exclude myocardial infarction.

A: AST non-specific for coronary disease rises within 18–36h.

B: CK-MB specific to heart muscle rises within 3–12h of onset of chest pain, reaches peak value in 24h and returns to base line in 48h. It is also present in other tissues (skeletal muscles, tongue, diaphragm, uterus) and trauma or surgery may lead to false positive results.

C: LDH starts rising in 24–36h after the onset of chest pain and peaks in 3 days, but is not sensitive or specific.

D: Myoglobin levels rise within 1–4h from onset of pain. They are highly sensitive but not specific.

For additional information, see *Emergencies in Cardiology*, 2nd edn, pp46–7, and the *Oxford Handbook of Acute Medicine*, 3rd edn, pp16–17.

→ www.nice.org.uk/nicemedia/live/12947/47938/47938.pdf

7. A ★

The features of acute severe asthma are respiratory rate >25/min, heart rate >100/min, inability to complete a sentence in one breath and PEFR 30–50% best or predicted. The classification of asthma denotes its severity and helps in determining the nature of treatment.

Fig. 3.26 shows PEFRs in normal adults.

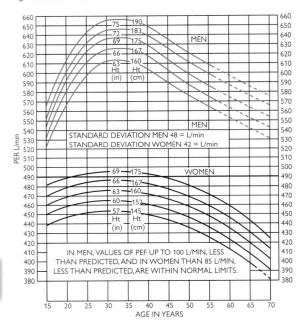

Table 3.2 Levels of severity of acute asthma exacerbations

Near-fatal asthma	Raised PaCO₂ and/or requiring mechanical ventilation with raised inflation pressures	
Life-threatening asthma	Any one of the following in a patient with severe asthma:	
	Clinical signs	Measurements
	Altered conscious level	PEF <33% best or predicted
	Exhaustion	SpO₂ <92%
	Arrhythmia	PaO₂ <8 kPa
	Hypotension	"normal" PaCO₂ (4.6–6.0 kPa)
	Cyanosis	
	Silent chest	
	Poor respiratory effort	

Acute severe asthma	Any one of: • PEF 33–50% best of predicted • Respiratory rate ≥25/min • Heart rate ≥110/min • Inability to complete sentences in one breath
Moderate asthma exacerbation	• Increasing symptoms • PEF >50–75% best or predicted • No features of acute severe asthma
Brittle asthma	• Type 1: wide PEF variability (>40% diurnal variation for >50% of the time over a period >150 days) despite intense therapy • Type 2: sudden severe attacks on a background of apparently well controlled asthma

Source: Adapted from British Thoracic Society and the Scottish Intercollegiate Guidelines Network (2009). *British Guideline on the Management of Asthma: A National Clinical Guideline*.

→ www.brit-thoracic.org.uk/Portals/0/Clinical%20Information/ Asthma/Guidelines/sign101%20revised%20June%2009.pdf

8. C ★

Steroids inhibit inflammation by preventing the release of pro-inflammatory mediators and cytokines from activated inflammatory cells.

A: Bronchial smooth muscle relaxation in asthma is achieved with β_2 agonists.

B: The bronchodilatory mechanism of the methylxanthines (e.g. theophylline, aminophylline) is unclear, but recent studies in COPD suggest they increase ventilatory drive rather than cause bronchodilation. They also increase mucociliary clearance and cardiac output, and inhibit the release of inflammatory mediators.

D: See C.

E: See B.

Marx JA, *et al.* (eds) (2010) *Rosen's Emergency Medicine: Concepts and Clinical Practice*, 7th edn. Philadelphia: Mosby/Elsevier, pp896–9.

9. E ★   OHEM, 4th edn → p112

The chest X-ray shows consolidation in the Rt. lower zone. Pneumonia is broadly classified as community-acquired, hospital-acquired, aspiration pneumonia and pneumonia in immunocompromised patients. Community-acquired pneumonia can be primary, secondary, or atypical. The commonest organism responsible for causing community-acquired pneumonia is *Streptococcus pneumoniae* (40% of cases). The other common ones are:

- *Haemophilus influenzae* (5%)
- *Mycoplasma* (11%)
- *Legionella* (4%)
- *Staphylococcus aureus* (2%)

For additional information, see the *Oxford Handbook of Acute Medicine*, 3rd edn, p167.

10. E ★   OHEM, 4th edn → p126

The most likely cause in this case is peptic ulceration as the patient is on NSAIDs because of the recent sprain. Aspirin or NSAID-induced erosive gastritis/oesphagitis in patients with above therapy may occur, but is less common (15%) than peptic ulcer (35–50%).

For additional information, see the *Oxford Handbook of Acute Medicine*, 3rd edn, p224.

→ www.sign.ac.uk/pdf/sign105.pdf

11. D ★   OHEM, 4th edn → pp126, 532

The most likely cause in this case is diverticular disease. The bloody stool with mucus and abdominal signs are indicative of diverticular disease, which is the most common cause of lower GI bleed in patients >60 years.

A: Angiodysplasia is the second most common cause after diverticular disease. The presentation is variable – from asymptomatic to frank melaena or haematochezia (passage of fresh or altered blood per rectum).

B: Colonic malignancy could be the source of bleeding but it less common than diverticular disease.

C: Colonic Crohn's disease may present as colitis with bloody diarrhoea associated with abdominal pain and systemic features such as fever and tachycardia.

E: Ischaemic colitis is the third most common cause after diverticular disease and angiodysplasia. The patients usually have left lower abdominal pain with loose stools and blood.

→ www.sign.ac.uk

12. C ★   OHEM, 4th edn → pp154–5

Rehydration and insulin therapy are the mainstays of treatment in DKA. In this situation, to start with give normal saline 1L in the first

30min, followed by 500mL of normal saline every half hourly with potassium for 8h. The dose of potassium should be titrated according to the serum potassium level (or check on arterial blood gas result for an initial guidance). Fluid replacement in elderly patients requires caution.

A: Colloids are reserved for hypotensive and oliguric patients and used to restore BP, which is then followed by the above regimen.

B: 5% dextrose solution is used following the initial treatment with normal saline and insulin after the blood glucose drops to <12mmol/L. It is not used before this stage for obvious reasons.

D: Although the total body potassium is low, the plasma potassium at this stage may be normal, low, or high. The potassium level drops with correction of acidosis and administration of insulin. Therefore, after the first litre of normal saline, unless the potassium is >5.5mmol/L, give at 20mmol/h with ECG monitoring, checking the levels regularly. Giving 40mmol/L potassium blindly in 30 min is dangerous.

E: The average fluid loss in DKA is 3–6L. Giving 1L of fluid in 4h in such patients will delay the recovery from acidosis causing serious consequences, such as development of shock and multiorgan failure.

13. A ★   OHEM, 4th edn → p61

Such patients fall ill rapidly. A careful assessment should be made when they come back to the ED even with trivial symptoms. A minimum investigation of full blood count should be done. This patient has a high possibility of neutropenic sepsis. Treat the patient in a side room with full barrier nursing. Take swabs from the site of the Hickman line and discuss with the microbiologist on call regarding choice of antibiotic and admitting the patient.

B: If there is an obvious sign of infection, the line may require removal, but it is not appropriate to change the line in the ED for asepsis.

C, D, and E: These are not appropriate actions in this case.

For additional information, see the *Oxford Handbook of Clinical Medicine*, 8th edn, pp346, 526.

14. A ★   OHEM, 4th edn → pp164–5

The patient has hyperkalaemia due to diabetic renal disease progressing to chronic kidney disease. The potassium level >6.5mmol/L should be treated urgently by IV calcium chloride 10mL 10% slow IV over 5min while monitoring the ECG. This antagonizes cardiac membrane excitability. This patient should also be given short-acting human soluble insulin 10 units with 50mL of 50% dextrose, which will increase the cellular uptake of potassium.

B: IV crystalloid is required if there is a volume deficit or acidosis.

C, D, and E: These may be given in the management of mild hyperkalaemia (K^+ 5.5–6mmol/L).

15. C ★

Exposure to air: Air must be expelled from the syringe otherwise the values will be inaccurate (pH increased and pCO_2 reduced) – as in this case.

A: Sample from vein: Compare the sample SaO_2 with the pulse oximeter value; usually they have a good correlation. In this case, they are same, so it is not a venous sampling error.

B: Delayed analysis of the sample may decrease pO_2, increase pCO_2, and decrease pH as blood continues to metabolize.

D: Ice use does not affect the values if the sample is analysed within 10min of collection.

E: Liquid heparin must be expelled before sampling. The small amount left inside the syringe is sufficient. Excess heparin will move the pO_2 value towards normal and because it is acidic it will lower the pH. Use a dry heparin syringe if available. But the commonest error is exposure to air.

For additional information, see *Emergencies in Respiratory Medicine*, p321.

16. D ★   OHEM, 4th edn → p177

The patient has developed allergic or urticarial reaction, generally attributed to an allergic antibody-mediated response to a donor's plasma proteins. Slow down or stop the transfusion temporarily and give chlorphenamine (IV or oral).

A: Hydrocortisone is rarely indicated in such a situation, but is often given in anaphylaxis alongside epinephrine.

B: This is not helpful.

C: This must be done if anaphylaxis is suspected (bronchospasm, cyanosis, hypotension), in which case stop the transfusion immediately and give epinephrine, and hydrocortisone IV. Anaphylaxis may be caused by anti-IgA in the donor's blood components (the patient is likely to have genetic IgA deficiency).

E: This is not required in allergic reactions, but it is required in cases of serious mismatch transfusion errors.

→ www.transfusionguidelines.org.uk

17. A ★   OHEM, 4th edn → p177

The patient has developed the most serious intravascular haemolytic transfusion reaction, which is most often due to clerical error. This must be avoided by correctly documenting and labelling blood tubes and forms combined with checking blood products prior to administration. The forms and the blood sample bottles *must* have patient's correct name, address, date of birth, NHS number (or ED number for foreign visitors), clinical details, the sender's name, signature, and date of request clearly documented. The form and the tubes must have the same information which should be handwritten at the patient's bedside by the person who is taking blood from the patient. Despite extensive training and assessment with regards to this issue, unfortunately, labelling errors still occur with similar frequency.

B: Two practitioners must check and confirm that the details on the traceability label on the blood component match the patient's full name, date of birth, and NHS number (wrist band if unconscious). Also ensure that the donation number, the patient's blood group/ RhD type all match. One person must not initiate the checks and the transfusion.

C: Antihistamines may be given prior to the transfusion if there is a previous history of mild urticarial/allergic reactions to blood or blood products.

D: Giving blood through a central line would not have avoided the reaction.

E: It is important to take a history of previous allergic reactions to blood or a blood product before starting the transfusion to minimize the risk of allergic reactions. But this would not avoid the haemolytic transfusion reaction mentioned in the scenario.

→ www.transfusionguidelines.org.uk

18. E ★

This patient has type 2 respiratory failure. A Venturi mask has a system to fit a valve (specific adaptor system) to deliver oxygen at different flow rates, at a reliable and specific FiO_2. The valves are different colours and deliver specific FiO_2 as follows:

- Blue 24%
- White 28%
- Orange 31%
- Yellow 35%
- Red 40%
- Green 60%.

To change the FiO_2, the valve needs to be changed, the FiO_2 cannot be increased or decreased by changing the oxygen flow. The required oxygen flow rate is written on the specific valves. This type of oxygen is specially used in the ED in type 2 respiratory failure and when accurate FiO_2 is needed. It reduces the risk of CO_2 retention in type 2 respiratory failure.

A: CPAP is a method to deliver oxygen with a tight fitting mask with special delivery equipment. It provides FiO_2 of around 80% and is useful in type 1 respiratory failure to correct hypoxia. It improves oxygenation by increasing mean airway pressure, thus increasing ventilation to collapsed alveoli. It also reduces the work of breathing. CPAP is commonly used in selected cases of pneumonia and left ventricular failure in the ED. This patient may subsequently require treatment with CPAP if he does not improve following standard therapy of oxygen delivery by Venturi mask, salbutamol and ipratropium bromide nebulizer, hydrocortisone IV, and antibiotics.

B: Hudson mask: This simple mask provides an FiO_2 of 50–60% when the oxygen is delivered at the rate of 5–8L/min. In the ED, this method is used frequently although it does not provide high flow or controlled oxygenation.

C: Nasal cannulae: The oxygen is delivered through prongs. If delivered at the rate of 2L/min, maximum FiO_2 achieved is about 28%, at 4L/min it is 35%, and 6L/min 45%. The flow rate is also dependent on the respiratory rate and amount of mouth breathing. This method of oxygen delivery may be used in the ED in COPD patients but it is difficult to ascertain the exact FiO_2, particularly when repeated blood gas analysis is required to monitor the effect of the therapy.

D: Reservoir bag is a mask with a bag hanging below. Oxygen delivery at the rate of 10–15L/min using this method provides a FiO_2 of 80–90%. This is the first line method for resuscitation in the ED of hypoxic patients without COPD. Start by inflating the bag by pressing on the valve. Put the mask on patient's face once the bag is fully inflated.

For additional information, see *Emergencies in Respiratory Medicine*, pp274–5, and *Emergencies in Critical Care*, p48.

19. A ★ ★   OHEM, 4th edn →p70

TIMI score for unstable angina/non-ST elevation myocardial infarction (NSTEMI) is determined by simply summing the number of risk factors (1 point for each) as shown below:

- Age ≥65 years
- ≥3 coronary risk factors (family history of coronary heart disease, hypertension, diabetes, current smoker and hypercholesterolaemia)

- Use of aspirin within 7 days
- Elevated cardiac markers
- ST segment deviation
- Prior angiographic evidence of coronary artery disease
- >2 angina events within 24h.

The combined risk of developing death, myocardial (re)infarction or recurrent severe ischaemia requiring revascularization within 14 days is as follows:

- Score 1 – 5%
- Score 2 – 8%
- Score 3 – 13%
- Score 4 – 20%
- Score 5 – 26%
- Score 6–7 – 41%.

A score of >3 often indicates high risk worthy of early intervention.

This patient has the following risk factors: age, coronary risk factors (diabetes, smoker, and hypertension). This gives him a score of 2.

The occurrence of ischaemic chest pain at rest without ST elevation is classed as unstable angina or NSTEMI. If the troponin is found to be elevated, it is defined as NSTEMI.

→ http://jama.ama-assn.org/cgi/content/abstract/284/7/835

Bassand J-P, Hamm CW, Ardissino D, Boersma E, Budaj A, Fernández-Avilés F, *et al.* (2007) Guidelines for the diagnosis and treatment of non-ST segment elevation acute coronary syndromes. The Task Force for the Diagnosis and Treatment of Non-ST-Segment Elevation Acute Coronary Syndromes of the European Society of Cardiology. *Eur Heart J* **28**:1598–660.

20. A ★ ★   OHEM, 4th edn → p113

The CURB-65 score is often used to judge the severity of pneumonia. Score 1 point for each of:

- Confusion
- Urea >7mmol/L
- Respiratory rate ≥30 breaths/min
- Low BP (systolic <90mmHg, diastolic ≤60mmHg)
- Age ≥65 years.

Patients with CURB-65 score ≥3 have severe pneumonia with a high risk of death. Patient with score of 0 or 1 are at low risk of death and may be suitable for home treatment.

→ www.brit-thoracic.org.uk/Portals/0/Clinical%20Information/
Pneumonia/Guidelines/MACAPrevisedApr04.pdf (go to Section 6)

21. D ★ ★   OHEM, 4th edn →p98

Pulse oximetry is a simple, rapid, safe, and non-invasive method of determining the SaO_2 of haemoglobin. It is based on the difference in light absorption between oxyhaemoglobin and deoxyhaemoglobin. But it does not provide information about ventilation (pCO_2). The accuracy of modern pulse oximeters is ±2% although they are less accurate in lower saturation ranges. When inaccuracies occur, the saturation is usually underestimated.

D: The effect depends on colour. Green and blue reduce the SaO_2 reading but red usually has no effect. Remove all varnish to obtain optimum reading.

A: The patient's BP is normal although hypotension may give erroneous readings because of poor tissue perfusion.

B: Though the patient probably has a chest infection, her arterial pO_2 is within normal limits and she is not hypoxic, therefore this is not the reason for her low reading.

C: Low haemoglobin (<5g/dL) may cause false readings. This patient has a normal haemoglobin level.

E: In hypothermia, the saturation reading is unreliable.

Other situations in which the pulse oximetry reading may be unreliable are:

- Excessive movement causing poor signal quality
- Carbon monoxide poisoning — falsely high reading as carboxyhaemoglobin reads as oxyhaemoglobin.
- Methaemoglobinaemia (falsely low when SaO_2 >85% and falsely high when <85%).

For additional information, see *Emergencies in Respiratory Medicine*, pp328–9.

22. B ★ ★   OHEM, 4th edn →p116

This patient has a right-sided pneumothorax, and since he is >50 years and also has chronic underlying lung disease, he should be admitted and treated with intercostal tube drainage. Needle aspiration in this case may be initially tried, but, even if successful, the patient should not be discharged. The other options are inappropriate.

Fig. 3.27 shows a flow chart for the management of spontaneous pneumothorax (taken from the British Thoracic Society 2010 guidelines on pleural disease).

MANAGEMENT OF SPONTANEOUS
PNEUMOTHORAX

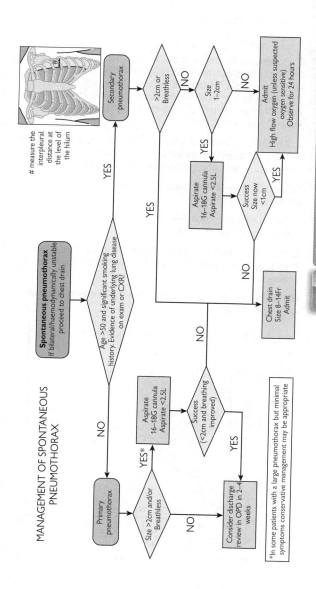

measure the
interpleural
distance at
the level of
the hilum

Spontaneous pneumothorax
If bilateral/haemodynamically unstable
proceed to chest drain

Age >50 and significant smoking
history. Evidence of underlying lung disease
on exam or CXR?

Secondary pneumothorax ← YES

Primary pneumothorax ← NO

Secondary pneumothorax branch:

>2cm or Breathless

— YES → Aspirate 16–18G cannula Aspirate <2.5L → Success Size now <1cm — YES → Admit High flow oxygen (unless suspected oxygen sensitive) Observe for 24 hours

— NO → Size 1–2cm

Size 1–2cm — NO → Admit High flow oxygen (unless suspected oxygen sensitive) Observe for 24 hours

Size 1–2cm — YES → Admit ...

Success Size now <1cm — NO → Chest drain Size 8–14Fr Admit

Primary pneumothorax branch:

Size >2cm and/or Breathless

— YES* → Aspirate 16–18G cannula Aspirate <2.5L → Success (<2cm and breathing improved) — YES → Consider discharge review in OPD in 2–4 weeks

— NO → Consider discharge review in OPD in 2–4 weeks

Success (<2cm and breathing improved) — NO → Chest drain Size 8–14Fr Admit

*In some patients with a large pneumothorax but minimal
symptoms conservative management may be appropriate

Medicine

111

→ www.brit-thoracic.org.uk/clinical- information/pneumothorax/
pneumothorax-guideline.aspx

23. B ★ ★   OHEM, 4th edn →p100

The patient has an acute exacerbation of COPD. In acute situations, because of alveolar hypoventilation, gas exchange is impaired leading to retention of carbon dioxide and respiratory acidosis. The kidneys try to compensate by retaining bicarbonate, but when patient reaches the stage of acute ventilatory failure, the pH is lowered, and the pCO_2 and bicarbonate are elevated.

A: This blood gas result indicates metabolic acidosis, where the pH is reduced, but the pCO_2 is normal with low standard bicarbonate and high negative base excess, often found in diabetic ketoacidosis.

C: This is a normal arterial blood gas analysis in someone who is breathing air.

D: The patient has hypoxia. This may be found in initial stages of asthma or a pulmonary embolism.

E: Respiratory alkalosis as the pH is high with low pCO_2, may occur in panic hyperventilation, initial stage of asthma, and pulmonary embolism.

Fig. 3.28 shows the acid–base nomogram in the interpretation of arterial blood gases.

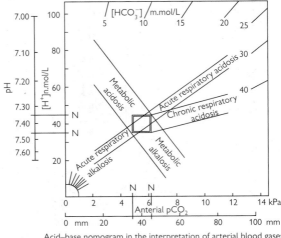

Acid–base nomogram in the interpretation of arterial blood gases

The patient has had a haemoptysis because of a chest infection. He is also septic. The urgent management would be putting him on high-flow oxygen, insertion of a wide bore cannula (which is already been done), taking blood for full blood count, inflammatory marker (CRP), and urea and electrolytes to check kidney function (because of sepsis), and culture and sensitivity. Sputum may also be collected for culture and sensitivity.

A: Antibiotics should be given IV after taking blood for culture and sensitivity.

B: Arterial blood gas is required if the patient is hypoxic, SaO_2 <92% on air. The lactate level may be checked as a part of sepsis management.

D: A portable chest X-ray may be arranged once the initial treatment is started.

E: ECG is not urgent, may be done after the above treatment is done.

25. C ★★

Hypovolaemic shock following blood loss in adults may be classified on the basis of clinical parameters into classes I–IV; the class equates to the percentage of approximate blood loss. There is no such grade of severity as Class V.

Table 3.3 Classification of haemorrhage severity

	Class I	Class II	Class III	Class IV
Volume of blood Volume (mL)	<750	750–1500	1500–2000	>2000
Blood loss in % of circulating blood volume	0–15	15–30	30–40	>40
Systolic BP	No change	Normal	Reduced	Very reduced
Diastolic BP	No change	Raised	Reduced	Very reduced/ unrecordable
Pulse (bpm)	Slight tachycardia	100–120	120 (thready)	>120 (very thready)
Respiratory rate	Normal	Normal	Raised (>20/min)	Raised (>20/ min)
Mental state	Alert, thirsty	Anxious or aggressive	Anxious, aggressive or drowsy	Drowsy, confused or unconscious

Adapted from Baskett PJF (1990). ABC of major trauma. Management of hypovolaemic shock. *BMJ* **300**:1453–7.

→ www.sign.ac.uk/pdf/sign105.pdf

Medicine

The simple ABCD^2 scoring system has been validated as a good predictor of future risk of stroke in patients presenting with TIAs in the ED. The criteria are as follows:

- Age: ≥60 years = 1 point
- BP: ≥160mmHg systolic and/or 90mmHg diastolic = 1
- Clinical features: unilateral weakness = 2; speech disturbance without weakness = 1; other = 0
- Duration of symptoms in minutes: ≥60mins = 2; 10–59 = 1; <10 = 0
- Diabetes: present = 1

Total score range: 0–7 points.

Risk of developing stroke in 48h:

- 6–7 points = 8%
- 4–5 points = 4%
- 0–3 points = 1%.

The patient in the scenario has a score of 6 points.

All such patients should be admitted for urgent investigation and management. Indicators for hospital admission are:

- ABCD^2 score ≥4
- Continuing symptoms or residual deficit
- >4 TIAs in the past 2 weeks
- Known severe stenosis in a vascular territory corresponding to the TIA symptoms
- Already taking antiplatelet therapy
- Suspected cardiac source of emboli (myocardial infarction, AF, valvular disease)
- Diagnostic uncertainty.

Rothwell PM, Giles MF, Flossmann E, Lovelock CE, Redgrave JN, Warlow CP, *et al.* (2005) A simple score (ABCD) to identify individuals at high early risk of stroke after transient ischaemic attack. *Lancet* **366**:29–36.

27. D ★★   OHEM, 4th edn →p150

All such patients should be asked about any changes to their seizure pattern. Causes of recurrence of seizures are: poor compliance with medication, alcohol or drug use, concurrent illness/infection, etc. Perform a detailed neurological examination and investigate for any intercurrent illness. After checking the vital signs, exclude hypoglycaemia by performing a bedside glucose test, and discharge patients who have fully recovered and have no concurrent illness or infection with advice about alcohol intake.

A: Admit the patient under the medical team if they have had a significant change to their seizure pattern or have a concurrent illness/infection that may have precipitated the seizure.

B: CT scan of the brain is required if the pattern of the seizure has changed or there is a suspicion of head injury.

C: There is no indication for changing the dose of the drug in the ED but the GP should be informed for follow-up.

E: This is not indicated.

28. B ★ ★   OHEM, 4th edn →p150

Some patients presenting with a first fit require an emergency CT scan of the brain to exclude serious underlying disease. The indications are: focal neurological deficit, fever, head injury, persistent headache, use of anticoagulants, history of AIDS, and prolonged post-ictal state.

A: After the brain scan admit the patient under the medical team to investigate and treat further as the patient has fever.

C: Antiepileptic medication should not be started following a first fit until the diagnosis of epilepsy is confirmed by a neurologist.

D: Patients who have fully recovered with no residual symptoms or signs and no suspicion of significant pathology may be discharged but all such patients must be followed up by their GP.

E: Subsequent neurological outpatient referral is mandatory (see C).

29. D ★ ★   OHEM, 4th edn →p178

The patient should be given IV morphine. The initial dose may be 5mg followed by further doses of 1–5mg if the patient is not responsive.

A and B: No specific test can detect a sickle cell crisis. But a full blood count should be done in all such patients and the present values compared with the previous visits. If the patient's haemoglobin level has decreased by more than 2g/dL from the baseline, a reticulocyte count should be obtained as a decrease of ≤3% in the count from the patient's usual value may denote an aplastic crisis.

C: A small number of patients with sickle cell disease attend the ED rather frequently and the ED staff tend to become suspicious of the patient's motives. All ED should have a protocol for staff to deal with such situations as there is a possibility of junior ED staff overlooking life-threatening complications due to this attitude. Patients should not be discharged without confirming absence of an acute crisis (which usually requires hospitalization).

E: Analgesia should be given promptly. The patient may be more cooperative after receiving an analgesic and allow a meaningful, detailed clinical examination of the abdomen.

For additional information, see the *Oxford Handbook of Acute Medicine*, 3rd edn, pp576–79, and the *Oxford Handbook of Clinical Medicine*, 8th edn, pp334–5.

Marx JA, *et al.* (eds) (2010) *Rosen's Emergency Medicine: Concepts and Clinical Practice*, 7th edn. Philadelphia: Mosby/Elsevier, pp1568–70.

30. B ★ ★ ★   OHEM, 4th edn → pp80–1

The patient has acute pericarditis. The inflammation in the pericardium may be idiopathic or of viral (Coxsackie, Epstein–Barr) or bacterial (tuberculous, acute rheumatic fever, pneumonia) origin. The other causes are uraemia, autoimmune diseases (systemic lupus erythematosus, rheumatoid arthritis), acute myocardial infarction, cardiac surgery, and chest radiotherapy. Such patients are relatively young with absence of signs of shock (cold/clammy skin, sweaty) as in acute myocardial infarction. The ECG in Fig. 3.7 shows generalized marked ST segment elevation and PR depression. Although it looks like an acute myocardial infarction, the reciprocal changes are absent. If there is doubt, confirm the diagnosis with an echocardiogram. Patients respond well to aspirin or NSAIDs taken orally (diclofenac 50mg three times per day or ibuprofen 400mg three times per day).

Aspirin is an antiplatelet drug that is very effective in primary and secondary prevention of ischaemic heart disease and stroke. It is given as a loading dose of 300mg followed by 75mg daily for life. In this case, aspirin is given because of its non-steroidal anti-inflammatory action in the dose of 600mg four times daily orally. Avoid indometacin as it reduces coronary flow.

A: There is no indication for giving antiplatelet drugs (these suppress platelet aggregation), which are given in ACS.

C: Pericardiocentesis is done if cardiac tamponade is suspected, the clinical features of which are:

- Tachycardia
- Reduced pulse pressure
- Hypotension
- Jugular venous distension – rises during inspiration
- Pulsus paradoxus – an exaggeration of normal physiology. The normal systolic BP difference between inspiration and expiration is increased to more than 10mmHg

- Muffled heart sounds and impalpable apex beats.

Echocardiography can confirm tamponade.

D and E: These are treatments for acute myocardial infarction.

For additional information, see the *Oxford Handbook of Acute Medicine*, 3rd edn, pp150–51, and *Emergencies in Cardiology*, pp204–6.

→ http://emedicine.medscape.com/article/156951-overview

31. D ★ ★ ★ OHEM, 4th edn → pp92–3

This patient has evidence of end-organ damage (left ventricular hypertrophy on ECG and renal impairment on blood test) and should be referred to a medical team for treatment as inpatient. The patient also requires investigations to elicit the reason for his chest pain, particularly to exclude ischaemic heart disease. The other options are inappropriate as the patient should not be discharged without adequate investigations.

ECG criteria of left ventricular hypertrophy are:

- Tall R waves >1.6mV in I, >2.6mV in $V_{4–6}$, deep S wave in III, aVR, and $V_{1–3}$
- R wave in V_5 + S wave in V_1 or V_2 >3.5mV
- Broad QRS >80ms
- Left axis deviation
- Impaired R wave progression $V_{1–3}$.

32. A ★ ★ ★ OHEM, 4th edn → p92

Patients with a diastolic pressure of more than 125mmHg or evidence of hypertensive encephalopathy should be referred to the medical team for admission. There is a significant risk of complications (cerebral and cardiac hypoperfusion) if the BP is reduced rapidly (except in acute myocardial infarction and aortic dissection). In many cases it is appropriate to commence additional oral antihypertensive therapy. While analgesics may be prescribed for the headache, it is not appropriate to change the antihypertensive agent in the ED. In hypertensive emergencies, aim to reduce the diastolic BP to 100–110mmHg in 2–4h and normalize in 2–3 days.

For additional information, see the *Oxford Handbook of Acute Medicine*, 3rd edn, pp134–35.

33. C ★ ★ ★ OHEM, 4th edn → p124

This patient has a Mallory–Weiss tear of the mucosa at the gastro-oesophageal junction following severe retching, which is common following ingestion of large bouts of alcohol.

117

These tears occur in the mucosa and submucosa of the stomach in 75% of affected individuals and at the gastroesophageal junction in 25%. Most Mallory–Weiss tears stop bleeding spontaneously.

A: Embolization by selective arteriography is done by introducing various substances into blood vessels to occlude them to prevent or reduce haemorrhage, reduce the blood supply to arteriovenous malformations, reduce the size of a tumour, etc. The procedure is performed by an interventional radiologist and is done when bleeding is continuous, that is, it has not shown signs of stoppage or there is re-bleeding after endoscopy.

B: Endoscopic cauterization or injection is indicated in actively bleeding lesions, non-bleeding visible vessels and, when technically possible, to ulcers with an adherent blood clot.

D: Surgical intervention or embolization may be attempted if the patient fails to respond to endoscopic treatment.

E: Tamponade with a Sengstaken–Blakemore tube is used in upper GI variceal bleeding, but increasingly such patients are treated by early endoscopy and band ligation (oesophageal varices) or injection of sclerosants (gastric varices).

For additional information, see the *Oxford Handbook of Acute Medicine,* 3rd edn, pp234–35.

→ www.sign.ac.uk (sign105)

34. C ★ ★ ★ OHEM, 4th edn →p146

The middle cerebral artery territory is most commonly involved in such situations. It causes marked motor and sensory disturbances on the contralateral side of the body, which are worse in the upper limbs and face than the lower limbs (as in this case). The hemianopia occurs on the same side as the lesion.

A: The anterior cerebral artery is less commonly affected than the middle cerebral artery and supplies the medial side of the frontal lobe, affecting its function when affected. Patients present with contralateral hemiplegia and hemisensory loss with weakness more pronounced in the lower limbs than the upper. The patient may have primitive grasp and sucking reflexes and bowel and bladder incontinence.

B: This occurs when the lenticulostriate arterioles, which arise from circle of Willis and supply deep structures such as the basal ganglia and internal capsule, are involved. These arteries are commonly involved in hypertensive patients and the condition is also known as 'small vessel disease'—degeneration of their walls. Patients may present with a pure motor or sensory stroke if the internal capsule is involved.

D: The typical consequence is an isolated hemianopia often sparing the macula as the occipital pole may receive blood supply from a branch of middle cerebral artery. There may be additional features of visual inattention and neglect.

E: In the presence of an adequate collateral circulation, occlusion of the vertebral artery may not produce any symptoms. If there is a lack of collateral circulation, the commonest artery involved is posterior inferior cerebellar, which supplies the lateral medulla. Typically there is ipsilateral Horner's syndrome (sympathetic pathway), ipsilateral cerebellar ataxia (cerebellar connections), ipsilateral loss of pain and temperature sensation on face and loss of the same in the contralateral limbs (spinothalamic tract), and nystagmus often to either side (cerebellar and vestibular nuclei).

Fig. 3.29a shows the occlusion of the cerebral arteries and Fig. 3.29b shows the circle of Willis at the base of the brain.

(a)

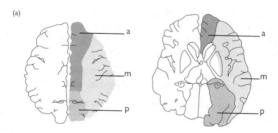

a = Anterior cerebral artery
m = Middle cerebral artery
p = Posterior cerebral artery

(b)

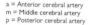

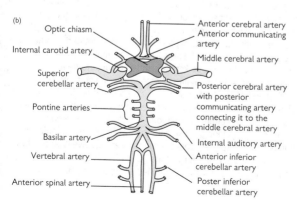

Optic chiasm

Internal carotid artery

Superior cerebellar artery

Pontine arteries

Basilar artery

Vertebral artery

Anterior spinal artery

Anterior cerebral artery
Anterior communicating artery

Middle cerebral artery

Posterior cerebral artery with posterior communicating artery connecting it to the middle cerebral artery

Internal auditory artery

Anterior inferior cerebellar artery

Poster inferior cerebellar artery

35. C ★ ★ ★ ★ OHEM, 4th edn →p157

This patient with COPD is in adrenal crisis. He has been on long-term steroids (COPD with bruises on the body) but has not been able to take his medication as he lay collapsed for an unknown period. Sudden withdrawal of medication may have precipitated the crisis. However, secondary infection may also be an additional precipitating factor. Adrenal crisis is a life-threatening condition that requires aggressive fluid resuscitation, hydrocortisone replacement, and treatment of the precipitating illness. After inserting a wide-bore cannula, blood samples should be taken for urea and electrolytes, random serum cortisol, and adrenocorticotropic hormone (ACTH). Treatment with dexamethasone 8 mg IV or hydrocortisone 100 mg IV should not be withheld while waiting for the blood results.

A: Broad-spectrum antibiotics may be prescribed as a further step after taking blood culture.

B: Give 50mL of 50% dextrose if the glucose level is below 3.5mmol/L.

D: As patient's SaO_2 is maintained at >90% on 31% FiO_2 and he has mild carbon dioxide retention on arterial blood gas testing, there is no urgency to increase the oxygen concentration. His acidosis may improve after treatment of the addisonian crisis.

E: There is no need to give sodium bicarbonate to treat acidosis, which may improve with crystalloid and steroid administration.

For additional information, see the *Oxford Handbook of Acute Medicine*, 3rd end, pp548–51.

36. E ★ ★ ★ ★ OHEM, 4th edn →p157

Adrenal crisis is uncommon but may occasionally present in the ED. The commonest cause is sudden withdrawal of regular steroid therapy either deliberately or inadvertently. In this case, the patient is unable to take her steroids because of vomiting. The characteristic feature of adrenal crisis is hypotension or shock out of proportion to the severity of the current illness. Other precipitating factors are uncommon but should be kept in mind to be able to treat the specific cause. After obtaining IV access, take a blood sample for cortisol and ACTH, start normal saline if patient is in shock, and give hydrocortisone sodium succinate 100mg stat. Take blood, urine, and sputum for culture if required to investigate for infection. Check capillary blood glucose and treat hypoglycaemia if indicated. If infection is suspected from the clinical features, give IV antibiotics after collecting samples for culture. The patient is not hypothermic (a body temperature of <35°C is defined as hypothermia).

37. A ★ ★ ★ ★ OHEM, 4th edn →p178

Acute chest syndrome is a common cause of hospitalization in sickle disease secondary to vaso-occlusive crisis. Such patients have a cough, breathlessness, fever, chest pain, and evidence of new infiltrates on the chest X-ray. The pathophysiology is not clear but acute chest syndrome is believed to be caused by sludging in the pulmonary microvascular network and pulmonary infarction. There is no definitive diagnostic test or treatment at present for this condition. The management is largely supportive in the form of analgesia, hydration, oxygenation, ventilation, and empirical antibiotics. Acute chest syndrome is the most common cause of death among patients with sickle cell disease.

B: Acute respiratory distress syndrome or acute lung injury occurs when the lung suffers an insult resulting in non-cardiogenic pulmonary oedema and hypoxia refractory to oxygen therapy. It is characterized by diffuse lung infiltrates, refractory hypoxia, reduced lung compliance, and respiratory distress. Causes are pneumonia, smoke inhalation, aspiration, sepsis, massive trauma, burns, acute pancreatitis, etc. For additional information, see *Emergencies in Respiratory Medicine*, pp114–15.

C: Congestive cardiac failure produces widespread pulmonary oedema on a background of underlying cardiac disease and/or associated risk factors.

D: Although the acute chest syndrome may be precipitated by infection, in pneumonia there is often a focal radiological heterogeneous opacity. See also the radiograph of a patient with pneumonia in Fig. 3.19.

E: The chest radiograph in pulmonary embolism is often normal, which may also be the case in acute chest syndrome. The presentation may be similar, but the diagnosis of pulmonary embolism may be suspected based on specific risk factors and appropriate investigations. With the background history of sickle cell disease, acute chest syndrome should be the first diagnosis to consider in this case.

For additional information, see *Emergencies in Respiratory Medicine*, pp250–1.

Marx JA, *et al.* (eds) (2010) *Rosen's Emergency Medicine: Concepts and Clinical Practice*, 7th edn. Philadelphia: Mosby/Elsevier, pp1568–70.

38. A ★ ★ ★ ★

The patient has hypercalcaemia of moderate grade (mild: 2.6–3.0mmol/L, moderate 3.1–3.4, severe >3.5). Rehydration with normal saline IV (0.9%) should be done. Aim for 3–6L in 24h. The goals of therapy are: rehydration, increased renal calcium elimination, treatment of primary disease, and reduction of osteoclastic activity. After rehydration, continue the saline infusion and give furosemide (this inhibits the resorption of calcium in the thick ascending loop of Henle) 40mg IV every 2–4h.

B: Calcitonin lowers calcium by reducing osteoclastic activity. It has the most rapid onset of action though it causes only a modest reduction in the calcium level. It is used in combination with bisphosphonate in severe hypercalcaemia where urgent reduction of calcium is necessary.

C: Dialysis is not a mode of primary management in hypercalcaemia.

D: Corticosteroids (glucocorticoids) are effective in hypercalcaemia caused by sarcoidosis, myeloma or Vitamin D intoxication. These drugs act by inhibiting the action of vitamin D.

E: Sodium pamidronate, a potent bisphosphonate, inhibits osteoclastic activity and is used in severe hypercalcaemia.

For additional information, see the *Oxford Handbook of Acute Medicine*, 3rd edn, pp544–45.

British National Formulary (2010) **59**:584–5.

39. D ★ ★ ★ ★

In patients in the terminal stages, particularly elderly patients with cancer, pain is the most feared preventable sequel. No patient should live or die with unrelieved pain. Therefore, give a combination of analgesics to make the patient comfortable. Take advice from the pain control team if available. Take a detailed history and examine the patient to understand the aetiology of the pain. Pain from local damage or nerve infiltration may be relieved with amitriptyline or gabapentin.

A: This is not appropriate, as the patient already has known disease.

B: The diagnosis of metastatic spinal disease is already known. There is no additional benefit of such request.

C: The advance directive of 'Do not attempt resuscitation' is only for cardiac arrest. No patient should die or live in pain.

E: This is an invasive procedure and may cause further distress. There are various other methods of giving analgesics that should be tried first.

For additional information, see the *Oxford Handbook of Clinical Medicine,* 8th edn, pp532–5.

40. C ★ ★ ★ ★

After receiving treatment, the patient's PEFR has improved to >75%, SaO$_2$ to 96%, and respiratory rate from 30 to 26 breaths/min. She may be discharged with medication after ensuring that she has received instructions on correct inhaler technique, adjustment of the therapy within the recommendations, peak flow measurement, and record keeping. She must attend her GP within the next 2 working days.

→ www.brit-thoracic.org.uk/Portals/0/Clinical%20Information/ Asthma/Guidelines/sign101%20revised%20June%202009.pdf (Go to page 99, Annex 3).

Extended Matching Questions

1. N ★   OHEM, 4th edn → p68

The patient has idiopathic costochondritis (Tietze's disease), in which pain occurs in upper costal cartilages. The onset may be sudden or gradual. The affected cartilage is swollen and tender. The condition is treated with non-steroidal analgesics. For additional information, see the *Oxford Handbook of Clinical Medicine*, 8th edn, p726.

Kinirons MT, Harold E (eds) (2005) *French's Index of Differential Diagnosis*, 14th edn. London: Hodder Arnold, p103.

2. L ★   OHEM, 4th edn → p68

Gradual onset of chest pain over the sternum which worsens on inspiration but with slight relief on bending forwards is suspicious of acute pericarditis. The pain is often described as 'sore', 'aching', 'stabbing', or 'sharp'. On auscultation, the presence of a pericardial rub, which is like 'feet crunching on snow' or 'saw like' in both systole and diastole, clinches the diagnosis. The pain is worse on lying flat because the visceral and parietal pericardia rub together, and so it is relieved by sitting up. The ECG may be normal in 10% of cases or may show widespread saddle-shaped ST segment elevation or PR depression.

For additional information, see *Emergencies in Cardiology*, pp204–6.

3. D ★   OHEM, 4th edn → p94

With the above history and hypertension as a risk factor, the most likely diagnosis is a dissecting thoracic aortic aneurysm. The pulses are absent or reduced in 20% of cases. The most common site for the dissection is in the ascending aorta or descending aorta just distal to the origin of the left subclavian artery. An abnormal aortic silhouette may be seen in up to 90% of chest X-rays. Dissection of the ascending aorta may present with clinical signs of aortic regurgitation (the above murmur) or cardiac tamponade.

For additional information, see *Emergencies in Cardiology*, pp190–3.

4. K ★   OHEM, 4th edn → p79

This patient has had a myocardial infarction with congestive cardiac failure. The three most common complications of this are arrhythmias, cardiac failure, and shock. Among the arrhythmias, ventricular extrasystole is the commonest, which may degenerate into VT and VF. A thorough clinical examination must be performed to look for signs of the complications. As a result of congestive cardiac failure, the patient has a raised respiratory rate and low SaO_2. In cardiogenic shock, the patient will have hypotension, cold and clammy skin, oliguria, and clouding of consciousness.

Kinirons M, Harold E (eds) (2005) *French's Index of Differential Diagnosis*, 14th edn. London: Hodder Arnold, p99.

5. M ★   OHEM, 4th edn → p22

The most likely diagnosis is pulmonary embolism. The initial presentation may be similar to that of acute myocardial infarction. A history of smoking, oral contraceptive use, immobilization for long period, etc. should be checked for and both legs examined for deep vein thrombosis. Elevation of jugular venous pressure is nearly always present. Gallop rhythm may be heard over the right ventricles. Peripheral cyanosis may also be found in this condition.

Kinirons M, Harold E (eds) (2005) *French's Index of Differential Diagnosis*, 14th edn. London: Hodder Arnold, p102.

6. J ★   OHEM, 4th edn → p90

Diagnosis: Atrial fibrillation with rapid ventricular response (some flutter waves in V_1 with 3:1 block).

The ECG shows acute AF. The patient is compromised with hypotension and probably pulmonary oedema. In such situations, regardless of the duration of onset, the patient should urgently receive oxygen, heparin (IV 5000–10 000IU) and synchronized DC shock (200–360J monophasic or 120–150J biphasic) under sedation or short general anaesthesia.

Acute AF (onset <48h) may be associated with ischaemic heart disease (33%), heart failure (24%), hypertension (26%), and valvular disease (7%). There are other cardiac (sick sinus syndrome, pericarditis, cardiomyopathy, etc.) and non-cardiac (sepsis, pulmonary embolism, thyrotoxicosis, hypovolaemia, etc.) causes. Clinical presentation may vary, some patients may be asymptomatic, some may present with palpitations, heart failure, angina, etc. A few may have life-threatening complications. In chronic AF, the fast ventricular rate may be due to fever, hypovolaemia, dehydration, or drug toxicity. In 50% of patients, the rhythm may revert back to normal spontaneously. Give oxygen, insert an IV cannula, send blood samples for full blood count, urea and electrolytes, and other relevant tests depending on the history and clinical examination. Do not give digoxin or adenosine (AV blocking drugs) in AF in Wolff–Parkinson–White syndrome as it may increase the rate of conduction through the accessory pathway causing cardiovascular collapse or VF and death.

For additional information, see the *Oxford Handbook of Clinical Medicine*, 8th edn, p91, and *Emergencies in Cardiology*, p162.

→ www.escardio.org/guidelines-surveys/esc-guidelines/GuidelinesDocuments/guidelines-afib-FT.pdf

→ www.nice.org.uk/nicemedia/live/10982/30055/30055.pdf

7. A ★   OHEM, 4th edn → p89

The ECG (Fig. 3.11) shows tachycardia with narrow QRS complex. This is often referred to as PSVT. Among patients with PSVT, the commonest form is AVNRT. The other form is AVRT, which occurs in Wolff–Parkinson–White syndrome, and is also benign unless it is associated with other structural heart disease. The ECG diagnosis of AVNRT is based on a regular narrow complex tachycardia in the range of 150–250bpm with P waves hidden behind the QRS complex or may appear as 'pseudo-R' waves at the end of each QRS complex. All cases of regular, narrow complex tachycardia are treated in the same way: initially with vagal manoeuvres (carotid massage, Valsalva manoeuvre, ocular pressure, etc.), followed by an adenosine IV bolus if the vagal manoeuvres are unsuccessful. Adenosine, a purine nucleoside, acts by temporarily blocking the conduction through the AV node, and has a very short half-life (10s); therefore it should be given rapidly followed by 10mL of rapid normal saline flush. Patients should be warned of the short-lived side effects of chest tightness, flushing, nausea, headache, dizziness, etc. If the patient is unstable with the rhythm, it should be treated with immediate synchronized electrical cardioversion.

→ For additional information, see *Emergencies in Cardiology*, pp170–3. http://www.resus.org.uk/pages/periarst.pdf

8. C ★

ECG diagnosis: complete heart block.

The patient has third-degree AV heart block or complete heart block. On the ECG (Fig. 3.12), there is complete dissociation between the P and QRS waves, i.e. every P wave is not followed by a QRS wave. The P and QRS waves are regular but independent of each other. The QRS complex may be wide or narrow. The patient is hypotensive and requires immediate treatment with atropine IV. Temporary transvenous pacing should be arranged if the QRS complexes are broad and heart rate is below 40bpm. The managment also includes stopping any rate-slowing medication or treating any precipitating causes such as acute myocardial infarction, drug overdose, and abnormal electrolytes.

For additional information, see *Emergencies in Cardiology*, pp146–9.

9. B ★   OHEM, 4th edn → p88

ECG diagnosis: broad complex tachycardia (ventricular tachycardia).

Broad complex tachycardia refers to arrhythmias with ventricular rate >100bpm and QRS complex duration >3 small squares (>0.12s). It originates from foci in ventricles or a supraventricular tachycardia if associated with bundle branch block. If the patient has previous history of cardiac disease (acute myocardial infarction, congestive heart failure, CABG, etc.), an ECG showing fusion beats (a supraventricular impulse conducted to the ventricle but coinciding/merging with the ventricular beat), capture beat (supraventricular beat conducted in the middle of the ventricular beat with normal sinus QRS morphology), AV dissociation or extreme left axis deviation, the rhythm is VT. If in doubt, treat as VT. If the patient is stable, attempt chemical cardioversion with amiodarone or lidocaine. Inform the anaesthetist for a short GA and prepare for back-up synchronized DC cardioversion.

For additional information, see *Emergencies in Cardiology*, pp178–83.

10. H ★   OHEM, 4th edn → p84

The most likely diagnosis in sinus bradycardia. It may be physiological (fit young patient at rest) or follow drug treatment (β-blockers, amiodarone etc.), systemic illness (hypothyroidism, hypothermia), or sinus node disease (sick sinus syndrome is the commonest in the elderly age group). The initial presentation may be asymptomatic or an incidental finding, or the patient may have fatigue, exertional dyspnoea, and, less commonly, syncope or presyncope (light-headedness, feeling of weakness, and fainting as opposed to syncope, which is fainting). On ECG, the heart rate is <60bpm (about 42bpm in this case) and P is followed by QRS. Immediate management involves assessment of the haemodynamic (BP, level of consciousness, signs of heart failure, etc.), thyroid, and electrolyte status. The patient does not require any emergency treatment, but if they are haemodynamically compromised or symptomatic, give atropine 1 mg IV. If the bradycardia does not reverse and is associated with symptoms, the patient may require a permanent pacemaker.

For additional information, see *Emergencies in Cardiology*, p140.

General feedback

Table 3.4 Vaughan Williams classification of antiarrhythmic drugs

	Mechanism of action	Examples
Class I		
IA	Sodium channel blockers	Quinidine
IB	Moderate prolongation of depolarization and conduction	Procainamide
IC	Minimally slow depolarization and conduction	Disopyramide
	Markedly slow depolarization and conduction	Lidocaine
		Phenytoin
		Flecainide
		Propafenone
Class II	β-blockers	
	Non-selective	Propranolol
	Cardio-selective (β$_1$)	Esmolol
		Atenolol
		Sotalol
Class III	Potassium channel blockers	Amiodarone
		Sotalol
Class IV	Calcium channel blockers	Verapamil
		Diltiazem
Miscellaneous	Slowing of AV conduction – both anterograde and retrograde paths of re-entrant circuit	Adenosine
	Inhibition of the ATPase enzyme, impairing the Na$^+$ and K$^+$ active transport across the cell membrane	Digoxin
	Controlling the ventricular response rate in narrow and broad complex tachycardia, used as second or third line of drug	Magnesium

From Vaughan Williams EM (1970) Classification of anti-arrhythmic drugs. In: Sandfte E, Flensted-Jensen E, Olesen KH (eds). *Symposium on Cardiac Arrhythmias.* Sweden, AB ASTRA: Södertälje, pp449–72.

11. J ★   OHEM, 4th edn → p116

The probable diagnosis in this patient is primary spontaneous pneumothorax, which most commonly occurs in men between 20 and 40 years of age. The pleuritic chest pain and breathlessness are of sudden onset, and 50% of patients may have had breathlessness for 2 days prior to presentation. Reduced expansion, absent or reduced air entry and hyperresonance on percussion are diagnostic of pneumothorax.

For additional information, see *Emergencies in Respiratory Medicine*, p164.

12. C ★   OHEM, 4th edn → p106

The patient has an acute exacerbation of asthma. The usual presenting symptoms are wheeze, cough, shortness of breath, and chest tightness. These symptoms may be variable, intermittent, and worse at night or in the early morning. The diagnosis is made on the basis of the combination of the presenting symptoms and signs and peak flow measurement.

For additional information, see *Emergencies in Respiratory Medicine*, p119.

13. D ★   OHEM, 4th edn → p112

The most probable diagnosis is consolidation in the left lower base. It is secondary to infection as suggested by the history and fever. The other clinical features may be reduced chest wall movement and dullness on percussion.

For additional information, see the *Oxford Handbook of Clinical Examination and Practical Skills*, p218.

14. K ★   OHEM, 4th edn → p105

The patient possibly has pleural effusion/empyema in the right base. A minimum of 400mL of fluid presence is required to elicit the clinical signs in a pleural effusion. The other associated sign may be reduced movement, but large effusions may displace the mediastinum (tracheal shift) to the opposite side.

For additional information, see *Emergencies in Respiratory Medicine*, p148.

15. B ★   OHEM, 4th edn → p110

The most likely diagnosis is emphysema. Chronic obstructive pulmonary disease, which is characterized by progressive airway destruction with little or no reversibility, includes emphysema and chronic bronchitis. Chronic bronchitis is defined clinically as cough, sputum production on most days for 3 months of 2 successive years. Emphysema is defined as pathologically enlarged air spaces distal to the terminal bronchioles with destruction of alveolar walls. The symptoms of both are cough, sputum (white), dyspnoea, and wheeze. The signs are tachypnoea, use of accessory muscles of respiration, hyperinflation, decreased crico-sternal distance (<3cm) reduced chest expansion, resonance or hyperresonance on percussion, and quiet breath sounds.

For additional information, see the *Oxford Handbook of Clinical Examination and Practical Skills*, p214.

16. I ★

The right lung is completely collapsed with shifting of the mediastinum to the left. This X-ray should not have been taken and the patient treated with needle thoracocentesis on the basis of clinical examination alone.

For additional information, see *Emergencies in Respiratory Medicine*, p164.

17. F ★

The chest X-ray in Fig. 3.16 show homogeneous opacity in the right lower zone with a meniscus-shaped upper border and extending to the chest wall. There is also an element of consolidation above the effusion.

For additional information, see *Emergencies in Respiratory Medicine*, p348.

18. A ★

The chest X-ray in Fig. 3.17 shows a ring-type shadow with a horizontal fluid level in the right upper zone (probable diagnosis is a lung abscess). The surrounding lung tissue shows diffuse opacity because of surrounding consolidation.

For additional information, see the *Oxford Handbook of Clinical Examination and Practical Skills*, p154, p738.

19. H ★   OHEM, 4th edn → p102

The chest X-ray in Fig. 3.18 shows severe pulmonary oedema with bilateral pleural effusion. The patient is in left ventricular failure. Note the interstitial horizontal lines (Kerley B lines) shadowing at the right base and peribronchial cuffing in the left mid zone.

For additional information, see *Emergencies in Respiratory Medicine*, p360.

20. C ★

The chest X-ray in Fig. 3.19 shows an opacity occupying the right lower zone and obscuring the right heart border completely. An air bronchogram is seen in the upper part of the shadow.

For additional information, see *Emergencies in Respiratory Medicine*, p360.

21. G ★   OHEM, 4th edn → pp230–2

60% of acute diarrhoea is due to viruses, of which the commonest in hospitals or institutions is the highly infectious norovirus. Symptoms include nausea, vomiting, diarrhoea, abdominal pains/cramps, myalgia, headache, malaise, chills, low-grade fever, or a combination of these symptoms. GI symptoms characteristically last 24–48h. Recovery is usually rapid thereafter. The duration of the illness is usually between 12 and 60h, with an incubation period of between 15 and 48h, and both staff and patients can become infected. This is not a notifiable disease.

Infections caused by rotavirus primarily occur in the winter months in infants and children, 6 months to 2 years of age.

22. B ★   OHEM, 4th edn → pp30–2

The most likely cause of the symptoms is campylobacter enteritis, caused by *Campylobacter* spp., the most common bacterial infectious agent in England and Wales. The source of infection is often undercooked poultry. The differential diagnosis includes infection with *Salmonella* spp. and *Shigella* spp., but in these the abdominal pain is less pronounced than in campylobacter infections. Diagnosis from the history alone may be difficult and requires stool culture for confirmation. Campylobacter organisms are small, spiral-shaped Gram-negative bacteria. The diarrhoea starts about 24–48h after the onset of fever and abdominal pain. Most patients recover within a week. This is a notifiable disease. Initial treatment is hydration.

→ www.patient.co.uk/doctor/Campylobacter-Enteritis.htm

23. C ★

The most probable causative organism is *C. difficile*, which should be considered in any patient who develops diarrhoea within 4 weeks of having antibiotics, oral or parental. *C. difficile* is an anaerobic, spore-forming Gram-positive bacillus that is normally found in the colon. It proliferates when the normal intestinal bacterial flora is reduced by antibiotic therapy and produces toxins; these toxins can be detected in the stool to make a definitive diagnosis. The clinical presentation is mostly mild, but may present with severe cramps, fever, dehydration, and blood in the stool. Mild cases can be treated with oral metronidazole. All affected patients require barrier nursing. This is not a notifiable disease.

24. D ★

The patient has traveller's diarrhoea; the most common pathogen is enterotoxigenic *E. coli*, which is transmitted via food and water in developing countries. The fever is unusual. Even in severe cases, the diarrhoea stops within 3–5 days.

A different strain of *E. coli* – serotype O157:H7 – produces haemorrhagic colitis, which may progress to haemolytic uraemic syndrome and/or thrombotic thrombocytopenic purpura. In this condition, diarrhoea is initially watery and then bloody, and is accompanied by severe abdominal cramps and vomiting. Fever if present is usually low grade, which differentiates the infection from Shiga toxin producing colitis. Uncomplicated *E. coli* infections resolve within 7–10 days. Haemolytic uraemic syndrome is notifiable.

25. K ★

The illness has a rapid onset because of the short incubation period of *Staphylococcus*. Staphylococci can multiply at room temperature in foods rich in protein and carbohydrate, such as ham, eggs, mayonnaise, potato salad, etc. The food poisoning is short-lived and the person recovers within 24h. Treatment is supportive. An antiemetic may be given to help control vomiting. Infection can be avoided by following strict personal hygiene among food handlers and refrigerating food that is not intended for immediate consumption. This is a notifiable disease.

For general feedback on this topic, see the Oxford Handbook of Acute Medicine, pp236–47.

→ www.hpa.org.uk/Topics/InfectiousDiseases/InfectionsAZ/
NotificationsOfInfectiousDiseases/ListOfNotifiableDiseases/

26. D ★   OHEM, 4th edn → p142

Such patients may present with syncope as a result of reduced cerebral perfusion on exertion or arrhythmias. Syncope is a sudden, transient loss of consciousness, with spontaneous recovery. This patient's ECG shows features of left ventricular hypertrophy and the clinical findings support the diagnosis of critical aortic stenosis.

For additional information, see Emergencies in Primary Care, pp134–5 and http://www.nice.org.uk/nicemedia/live/13111/50452.pdf.

Medicine

Aortic dissection may present in hypertensive patients with sudden onset of severe, sharp, tearing, or stabbing pain, maximal at onset, in the anterior or posterior chest. Syncope occurs in about 10% of patients. Dissection may spread proximally causing aortic regurgitation (which this patient has), coronary artery blockage, and cardiac tamponade. It may spread distally, blocking the origin of various arteries and causing symptoms such as neurological deficit with chest pain. Such patients are often hypotensive on presentation. The presentation may mimic that of acute myocardial infarction, and requires a high index of suspicion.

28. H ★   OHEM, 4th edn → p122

Pulmonary embolism may present with syncope. Previous cancer treatment or surgery may precipitate sudden-onset pulmonary embolism. In the ED, patients with pulmonary embolism may present with dizziness, syncope, shortness of breath, malaise, and pain. Around 50% of such patients may not have risk factors for pulmonary embolism. A typical presentation is worsening shortness of breath over a couple of days, which forces the patient to seek advice. The onset may be sudden in 50% of cases. The pain may be vague and is often only on one side. Central chest pain is often cardiac in origin, or has other causes but rarely pulmonary embolism.

29. A ★   OHEM, 4th edn → p546

AAA rupture is common in middle-aged and elderly people, and is responsible for a large number of deaths. The presentation is variable. The classic history is of central abdominal pain and lower back pain in a patient with a known aneurysm. The typical triad of symptoms is described as pain, hypotension, and a pulsatile mass. Many patients have one or two of these features although some will have none of them. The pain is typically sudden in onset and severe in nature. It may be felt in the flank and radiate to chest, thigh, and inguinal area.

For additional information, see *Emergencies in Primary Care*, p52.

30. G ★   OHEM, 4th edn → p68

This man has an acute myocardial infarction (posterior-lateral type), which excludes all other options. Subarachnoid haemorrhage may have an ECG finding of ST-T wave changes, U waves, and prolonged QT interval, but it usually presents with headache and syncope. The ECG findings may confuse a clinician and may result in an erroneous diagnosis of acute cardiac ischaemia, hence a careful history is important.

For additional information, see the *Oxford Handbook of Acute Medicine*, 3rd edn, pp12–13.

Medicine

31. M ★   OHEM, 4th edn → p128

The pain of a tension headache may be continuous, pressing or tight, band-like in nature usually in the occipital or bilateral temporal area. Unlike migraine physical exertion does not worsen the pain and the other symptoms associated with migraine including photophobia, nausea, vomiting, etc. are absent usually. The diagnosis is based on absence of features that would suggest other organic pathology. Anxiety or depression may coexist. Despite tension headaches, patients usually are able to carry on with their usual activities and sleep. Simple analgesia with paracetamol or NSAIDs is adequate to control pain.

32. K ★   OHEM, 4th edn → p130

Subarachnoid haemorrhage should be considered in any patient with a sudden onset of severe headache. The onset may be described as 'a blow to the head', 'the worst headache of my life', 'worst ever' headache, etc. The onset may be associated with exertional activities such as exercise, coughing, or sneezing, or sexual intercourse in 20% of cases. About 75% of patients may have associated nausea and vomiting. More than 50% of patients may have features of meningism (headache, neck stiffness, and photophobia). Such patients require CT scan of the brain to establish the diagnosis. If the scan is normal (in about 5%), they should undergo a lumbar puncture at least 12h after the onset of the headache for detection of xanthochromia in the CSF. Xanthochromia may take up to 12h to appear in the CSF after the initial bleeding.

33. F ★   OHEM, 4th edn → p134

Giant cell arteritis or temporal arteritis is a systemic inflammation (segmental granulomatous panarteritis) of small- and medium-sized arteries. It is rare <50 years. The mean age is 70 years with a female:male ratio of 2:1. Headache is the most common initial presentation (90%), which may be sharp or throbbing/aching type, and may be localized to the temporal area or generalized. Other likely features include night sweats, low-grade fever, jaw claudication, visual symptoms, early morning shoulder girdle stiffness and muscular aches (polymyalgia). On physical examination, temporal artery tenderness is present in about 85% of cases and scalp tenderness in 75%. The artery may be pulseless or thickened. The temporal artery should be best palpated lightly in front and slightly superior to the tragus. On investigation, the ESR is >50mm/1st h in 95% of cases, however, a normal ESR does not exclude the diagnosis. The risk of missing the diagnosis is subsequent blindness due to ischaemic optic neuropathy through involvement of the ophthalmic artery. If giant cell arteritis is suspected start hydrocortisone 200mg IV or prednisolone 40mg orally and arrange for a urgent temporal artery biopsy by referring to a neurologist.

34. H ★ OHEM, 4th edn → p228

This patient has meningitis. The classic picture of headache, neck stiffness, vomiting, fever, drowsiness, and photophobia suggest the diagnosis. Meningitis may be difficult to diagnose in the early stages because of the vague symptoms. Once suspected, after taking blood for routine investigation and culture, and starting antibiotics, arrange an urgent CT scan of the brain.

35. L ★

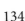

Patients often have headache, sleepiness, intellectual sluggishness, personality change, fluctuating level of consciousness, and unsteadiness, and may present with seizures and/or localizing neurological signs. Most subdural haemorrhages are caused by trauma which is *often forgotten as it was either trivial and/or a long time ago* (up to 9 months). The diagnosis can be confirmed on a CT scan of the brain.

36. J ★ OHEM, 4th edn → p152

The patient probably has type 1 diabetes (injection marks on abdomen). Hypoglycaemia must be excluded in any patient who presents with coma, altered behaviour, and neurological symptoms or signs. The normal plasma glucose level is 3.6–5.8mmol/L. Hypoglycaemia can present in various ways: sweating, pallor, tachycardia, trembling, irritability, violent behaviour, seizures, etc. Pupils of 3mm and a respiratory rate of 18 breaths/min exclude opioid poisoning, in which the pupils are more constricted and the respiration rate is also slower.

37. I ★ OHEM, 4th edn → p139

Coma with small pupils (1–2mm) and respiratory depression (<12 breaths/min) suggests opioid poisoning. Clear and maintain the airway. If the respiration is severely depressed, ventilate with a bag, valve, and mask or an endotracheal tube. IV naloxone should be given. The initial dose should be 0.8mg (2mL), which may be repeated if necessary every 2–3 min. In any patient with unexplained coma or coma without lateralizing signs, give a therapeutic trial of naloxone IV, observing any change in the conscious level. This patient's GCS score is 3 with spontaneous breathing.

38. A ★   OHEM, 4th edn → pp138–41

This patient is unconscious with GCS score of 6/15 and a dilated right pupil and upgoing plantars. She is also developing increasing intracranial pressure with slowing of her heart and respiratory rate and increasing BP. The most likely diagnosis is an intracranial bleed. Airway patency is the priority and this should be cleared and protected immediately.

Medicine

39. D ★

This patient has hyperosmolar non-ketotic coma (Hyperosmolar hyperglycaemic state), which occurs in elderly patients with type 2 diabetes. The mortality is higher than for ketoacidosis. Often there is no history of diabetes and such patients may present with severe dehydration, coma, or impaired conscious level. Coma is usually associated with an osmolality >440mOsm/kg. The mainstay of treatment is protection of the airway, oxygen, rehydration, and insulin therapy. Fluid replacement should be done more cautiously in the elderly.

For additional information, see the *Oxford Handbook of Acute Medicine*, 3rd edn, pp524–25.

40. B ★   OHEM, 4th edn → p228

This patient has meningitis and probably septic shock. Immediately after initial airway, breathing, and circulation management, and a glucose test, antibiotic IV should be given before arranging a CT scan. Lumbar puncture should be avoided as the first line of investigation because it may result in uncal coning if there are features of intracranial hypertension. CT, however, will not exclude increased intracranial hypertension, but is done to exclude space-occupying lesions and hydrocephalus.

41. I ★★   OHEM, 4th edn → p90

Diagnosis: AF with rapid ventricular response.

The ECG shows AF with rapid ventricular response. In the background of ischaemic heart disease, hypertension, and diabetes, patients often have chronic heart failure. They may have an acute exacerbation because of lack of compliance, uncontrolled hypertension, infection, arrhythmias, inadequate therapy, myocardial infarction, fluid overload, etc. Treatment aims to reduce the preload and afterload with a combination of diuretics and vasodilators. Make the patient sit up and give oxygen therapy to achieve an SaO_2 >95%. The patient will also require investigations to find out the cause of the AF and start appropriate treatment.

For additional information, see *Emergencies in Cardiology*, pp68–91.

42. F ★ ★   OHEM, 4th edn →p102

ECG diagnosis: LBBB.

The ECG shows LBBB with a heart rate of 90bpm. The features of LBBB are: broad QRS >0.12s because of delay in septal and left ventricular activation, an initial Q in V_1, R-S-R' pattern in V_6 (QRS is W shaped in V_1 and M shaped in V_6) and complete loss of R waves in V_{1-4} with ST elevation and peaked T waves. The patient is in acute-on-chronic heart failure. He requires oxygen, furosemide 40mg IV (which takes about 5–10min to act), morphine 2.5–10mg IV titrated (to reduce anxiety and which also acts as a vasodilator in such situation). Loop diuretics inhibit sodium resorption from the renal filtrate in Henle's loop resulting in increases in renal salt and water excretion. It reduces plasma volume, thus decreasing preload and pulmonary congestion in patients with volume overload. The patient may also require a GTN spray in addition to the loop diuretic. Patients with abrupt acute pulmonary oedema who do not have underlying chronic heart failure may have low plasma volume at presentation and should not be given diuretics.

For additional information, see *Emergencies in Cardiology*, pp68–91.

43. L ★ ★

ECG diagnosis: Prolonged QT interval (QT 536 s, QTc 569 s)

The patient has prolonged QT interval. The cause may be congenital, hypokalaemia, hypomagnesaemia, or drug induced (quinidine, flecainide, amiodarone, sotalol, amitriptyline, etc.). The main risk of a prolonged QT interval is of degenerating into polymorphic VT. Therefore, after the initiation of treatment for acute heart failure, investigations should be done to find out the cause of the arrhythmia and appropriate treatment started. After the initial treatment for acute heart failure with oxygen, morphine, and diuretics, if the patient is not responding, an IV infusion of vasodilator (nitrites) should be started if the systolic BP is >110mmHg. At lower doses, nitrates are primarily venodilators and effectively decrease pulmonary artery occlusion pressure. At higher doses, IV GTN also causes arteriolar dilation, which decreases BP and afterload. Thus, myocardial pump function is improved while myocardial oxygen demands are decreased.

For additional information, see *Emergencies in Cardiology*, p344.

44. E ★ ★   OHEM, 4th edn → p102
ECG diagnosis: Sinus tachycardia.

The patient has sinus tachycardia (heart rate around 105bpm). The BP is below 90mmHg, nitrites cannot be used and furosemide should be used cautiously. A cautious fluid challenge may be given as 100–200mL of saline as a bolus or 250mL saline over 10min. If the clinical situation does not improve, the patient may require inotropic support (dobutamine/dopamine). Arterial blood gases and chest X-ray should be done with other blood tests to explore the cause of heart failure.

For additional information, see *Emergencies in Cardiology*, p158.

45. D ★ ★   OHEM, 4th edn → pp102, 90
ECG diagnosis: Atrial flutter with rapid ventricular rate (3:1 block = the atrial rate is around 300bpm).

The patient is probably in acute-on-chronic heart failure. Continuous positive airway pressure is very effective in left ventricular failure. It increases functional residual capacity, thus increasing the effective alveolar surface area and improving the oxygenation. It also reduces the work of breathing and left ventricular preload, and improves ejection fraction. If the patient does not respond to conventional initial management of acute heart failure, continuous positive airway pressure should be considered.

For additional information, see *Emergencies in Cardiology*, pp10, 72.

General feedback
Fig. 3.30 shows a flow diagram for the management of heart failure (from the *Oxford Handbook of Clinical Medicine*, 8th edn, p813).

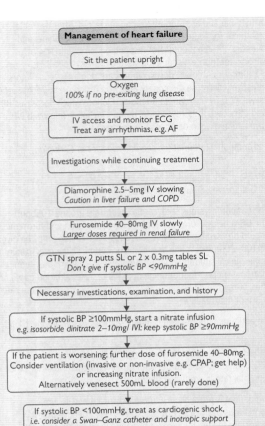

Management of heart failure

Sit the patient upright

↓

Oxygen
100% if no pre-exiting lung disease

↓

IV access and monitor ECG
Treat any arrhythmias, e.g. AF

↓

Investigations while continuing treatment

↓

Diamorphine 2.5–5mg IV slowing
Caution in liver failure and COPD

↓

Furosemide 40–80mg IV slowly
Larger doses required in renal failure

↓

GTN spray 2 putts SL or 2 × 0.3mg tables SL
Don't give if systolic BP <90mmHg

↓

Necessary investigations, examination, and history

↓

If systolic BP ≥100mmHg, start a nitrate infusion
e.g. isosorbide dinitrate 2–10mg/ IVI: keep systolic BP ≥90mmHg

↓

If the patient is worsening: further dose of furosemide 40–80mg.
Consider ventilation (invasive or non-invasive e.g. CPAP; get help)
or increasing nitrate infusion.
Alternatively venesect 500mL blood (rarely done)

↓

If systolic BP <100mmHg, treat as cardiogenic shock,
i.e. consider a Swan–Ganz catheter and inotropic support

Note:
- If failure to improve, reassess and consider alternative dianoses,
  e.g. hypertensive heart failure, aortic dissection, pulmonary embolism,
  pneumonia.
- CPAP (5–10mmHg) in dyspnoeic patients (if no ↓BP or emergent need
  for intubation) can reduce the need for intubation, and possibly
  in-hospital mortality.
- Consider IV nitrate therapy for patients with dyspnoea.

→ www.escardio.org/guidelines-surveys/esc-guidelines/
GuidelinesDocuments/guidelines-HF-FT.pdf

O'Brien JF, Falk JL (2010) Heart failure. In: Marx JA, *et al.* (eds)
Rosen's Emergency Medicine: Concepts and Clinical Practice, 7th
edn. Philadelphia: Mosby/Elsevier, pp1037–53.

CHAPTER 4

POISONING

'Never take the antidote before the poison'

Latin proverb

EDs in the UK see a significant number of patients (347 per 100 000/year and ever-increasing) with acute overdose of drugs. Most of them are ingested orally, but other modes of intake can be used, such as IV and nasal. Sometimes it is not uncommon to see a patient presenting themselves to the ED feeling unwell after having ingested packets of Class I drugs to transport across continents. Another group of patients include those who present themselves after self-harming with a knife or blade on their wrists, arms, abdomen, or other parts of the body. These patients may have a previous history of drug overdose.

Management of situations such as those described above requires both a generalized approach and specific actions against each drug involved. The common antidotes are covered in this chapter and advice is available in all EDs through the NPIS (<WEB>www.toxbase.org) to deal with such emergencies, particularly with the treatments of unusual poisons. I encourage all the junior doctors to use the website for all the poison cases presenting to the ED to help build up confidence while treating them. Readers should note though that the URLs provided in this chapter can be accessed only by foundation and more senior doctors as the NPIS does not provide usernames and passwords to medical students.

The priorities in the management of poisoned patients are similar to other ED presentations (ABCDE). Most of these patients require supportive therapy for recovery. Some poisons have specific antidotes which could be life-saving and are to be administered straightway. The initial assessment should be able to indicate whether or not the patient has been exposed to a specific poison for which an antidote is available. Hypoglycaemia must be excluded in every patient who presents with a low GCS score or convulsions by performing a capillary blood glucose by the bedside. A patient with respiratory depression, low GCS, and constricted pupils should be given *naloxone* while preparations are made to secure the airway. The recognition of such a pattern sometimes may direct the treating clinician towards a specific poison immediately, so that treatment with a definitive antidote can be given without delay. After the initial stabilization of a critically ill patient and the institution of the specific antidote (if indicated), a detailed drug overdose history and physical examination are required.

Inseparable from the presentation of drug overdose/self-harm is the underlying mental health status. For a junior doctor, once the medical aspect of the patient is taken care of, and the patient's clinical condition is stabilized, the care is never complete without an evaluation of the mental health status of such patients. The most important issue to focus on in the history is whether the overdose attempt was suicidal. Often vital clues can be obtained by collecting relevant information from the paramedics, relatives, or previous medical records. Therefore, almost every case requires the attention of a mental health specialist. If someone is seriously suicidal, this may be an emergency and the patient may require admission to the mental health ward after treatment for the overdose. Other patients may be seen and discharged from the ED after a consultation with a mental health liaison nurse, or they may be attended to in the community. ■

SINGLE BEST ANSWERS

1. A 22-year-old woman says she has taken about 40 tablets of paracetamol 3h ago. Her heart rate is 110bpm, BP 110/80mmHg, and respiratory rate 22breaths/min. Which is the *single* most appropriate initial management? ★

A Giving activated charcoal

B Giving *N*-acetylcysteine

C Inducing vomiting

D Performing gastric lavage

E Waiting for the 4h paracetamol level

2. A 30-year-old woman says she has taken about 34 tablets of paracetamol about 12h ago. She is now unwell. Her heart rate is 120bpm, BP 112/78mmHg, and respiratory rate 20breaths/min. Which is the *single* most important initial management? ★

A Discussing with the liver transplant unit

B Giving acetylcysteine immediately

C Giving activated charcoal immediately

D Referral for psychiatric assessment

E Waiting for the 4h paracetamol level

3. A 32-year-old man has been brought from the psychiatry unit after allegedly swallowing foreign bodies. He is physically well. His X-ray is shown in Fig. 4.1.

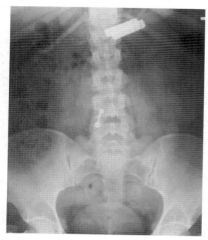

Which is the *single* most appropriate immediate management? ★

A Admitting to medical ward for observation

B Arranging endoscopic removal

C Arranging whole bowel irrigation

D Repeating X-ray in 2 days

E Using magnet for removal

4. A 20-year-old woman says she has taken about 40 tablets of paracetamol over the past 3 days. She is now unwell and has vomited a few times. Her heart rate is 110bpm, BP 110/80mmHg, and respiratory rate 22breaths/min. The blood test results are follows:

```
Sodium 146mmol/L; Potassium 3.5mmol/L; Urea
5.6mmol/L; Creatinine 115µmol/L; Albumin
32g/L; Bilirubin 52µmol/L;
ALT 2560IU/L; Alkaline phosphatase 230IU/L;
Gamma glutamyl transpeptidase 126IU/L;
pH 7.3; INR 4.0; Lactate 4.2mmol/L;
Paracetamol 190mg/L.
```

Which is the *single* most likely chemical compound responsible for these findings? ★ ★

A NAPQI

B *N*-para-acetylaminophenol

C *N*-para-acetylaminophenol glucuronide

D Para-acetylaminophenol sulfate

E Para-aminophenol

5. A 36-year-old woman has taken about 28 tablets of paracetamol 6h ago. She has been drinking a bottle of vodka and a couple of pints of lager every day for the last few years. She feels nauseous and has vomited few times.

```
Sodium 144mmol/L; Potassium 3.8mmol/L; Urea
5.6mmol/L; Creatinine 86µmol/L;
Albumin 30g/L; Bilirubin 15µmol/L;
ALT 30IU/L; AST 32IU/L; Alkaline phosphatase
280IU/L; Gamma glutamyl transpeptidase
126IU/L; Paracetamol 80mg/L.
```

Which is the *single* most appropriate immediate management? ★ ★ ★ ★

A Discussing with liver transplant unit

B Giving acetylcysteine

C Giving fresh frozen plasma

D Giving vitamin K injection

E Repeating the blood tests

6. An 18-year-old man had a bottle of vodka and 10 pints of lager while celebrating his birthday with friends. His GCS score is 8. His pulse is 100bpm, respiratory rate 8breaths/min, BP 90/70mmHg, and temperature 35°C. His finger prick glucose test result is 3.9mmol and blood ethanol concentration 310mg/dL. Which is the *single* most appropriate immediate management? ★ ★ ★ ★

A Arranging endotracheal intubation

B Giving activated charcoal

C Giving immediate glucagon

D Giving thiamine IV

E Performing gastric lavage

Poisoning

7. A 64-year-old man has been brought to the ED from a caravan site in the early hours of the morning after being found unconscious in his bed. His accompanying spouse has also been having headaches and nausea. There is no history of injury. After initial management by the ambulance crew, he is better and his GCS score is now 14. He has a headache and nausea, but a normal neurological and cardiovascular examination. Which is the *single* most important immediate management? ★ ★ ★ ★

A Endotracheal intubation

B Hyperbaric oxygen therapy

C IV crystalloid

D Non-invasive ventilation

E Oxygen with a tight-fitting mask

EXTENDED MATCHING QUESTIONS

Management of poisoning

For each of the following scenarios, choose the *single* most definitive management from the list of options below. Each answer may be used once, more than once, or not at all.

A Acetylcysteine

B Activated charcoal

C Atropine

D Flumazenil

E Gastric lavage

F Glucagon

G Glucose

H Naloxone

I Oxygen

J Sodium bicarbonate

1. A 23-year-old woman has been brought to the ED by blue light ambulance after having a respiratory arrest. She apparently injected herself with a drug. Her heart rate is 90bpm and BP 103/70mmHg.

2. An 80-year-old woman while having her shoulder reduced in the emergency department has been given 2mg of morphine and three aliquots of 5mg of midazolam intravenously within 5min. After the reduction, she is responding to pain. Her heart rate is 60bpm, BP 130/90mmHg, respiratory rate 10breaths/min, and oxygen saturation of 86%.

3. A 32-year-old woman has taken an unknown number of amitriptyline tablets. She is opening her eyes on vocal command, withdrawing on painful stimulus, and is making incomprehensible sounds. The ECG shows a heart rate of 122bpm, PR interval 0.28s, and QRS 0.2s. The pH is 6.9, pO_2 28kPa on 40% oxygen, pCO_2 4.0kPa, bicarbonate 19mmol/L, and base excess −6.

4. A 76-year-old man has taken 30 atenolol tablets, one of his regular medications. He is feeling unwell, and his heart rate is 54bpm and BP 110/70mmHg.

5. A 28-year-old woman has taken an unknown number of paracetamol and aspirin tablets about 5h earlier. Her paracetamol and salicylate levels are 54mg/L and 510mg/L, respectively.

POISONING
ANSWERS

Single Best Answers

1. E ★   OHEM, 4th edn → pp192–5

As the patient's history is often unreliable, the NPIS advises to measure the paracetamol level after 4h of ingestion and then give N-acetylcysteine if indicated. However, the drug should be given before the paracetamol levels are available if patients present 8h or more after the ingestion. N-acetylcysteine is most effective if given within 8–12h of ingestion. Charcoal should be given only if the patient has taken 12g or more than 150mg/kg body weight (whichever is smaller) of paracetamol and presents within 1h of ingestion. Induction of vomiting or gastric lavage does not have any role.

→ www.toxbase.org/Chemicals/Management-Pages/Paracetamol---adult-management--4h/

2. B ★   OHEM, 4th edn → p193

This patient's treatment plan falls under category of patients presenting 8–24h after paracetamol ingestion. The patient should be given acetylcysteine immediately without waiting for the paracetamol level as she has probably taken more than >12g of paracetamol. Usually it takes 2–3 days to affect the liver and grossly abnormal liver function tests should be discussed with the liver transplant unit. Activated charcoal is only effective if the patient has taken the overdose within the past 1h.

→ www.toxbase.org/Chemicals/Management-Pages/Paracetamol---management-8-to15-h/

3. D ★

The patient has ingested two batteries, (Fig. 4.1). They are in the stomach and should pass spontaneously through the rectum but this may take up to 2 weeks. If the patient remains asymptomatic, there is no need of active intervention and a repeat X-ray may be done after 2 days to check that the batteries have moved out of the pylorus and have not disintegrated. Gut decontamination is not required. Magnet removal is only tried in case of button batteries that have got stuck in the oesophagus.

The metal object in front of L3/4 in Fig. 4.1 is an artefact (umbilical piercing).

→ www.toxbase.org/Poisons-Index-A-Z/B-Products/Batteries/

4. A ★★

This patient has acute hepatic failure, renal failure, and acidosis following ingestion of paracetamol. Once paracetamol is absorbed completely within 4h, 90% of the drug is excreted after being metabolized in the liver. It is metabolized in the liver in three ways: conjugation with glucuronide, conjugation with sulfate, and oxidation through the cytochrome P_{450} oxidase system. The oxidation of paracetamol by the cytochrome system results in formation of highly cytotoxic intermediary compound, NAPQI, which then combines rapidly with glutathione forming non-toxic compounds and is excreted in urine. When glutathione supply is exhausted, the excess NAPQI binds to the hepatocytes causing toxicity.

B: *N*-para-acetylaminophenol is the chemical name of paracetamol from where the name paracetamol is derived. Para aminophenol is a precursor of paracetamol in the process of its manufacturing.

C and D: These are intermediate metabolites in the metabolism of paracetamol in the body but excreted in urine without causing any harm to the liver.

Hendrickson RG, McKeown NJ. Acetaminophen. In: Marx JA, *et al.* (eds) (2010) *Rosen's Emergency Medicine: Concepts and Clinical Practice*, 7th edn. Philadelphia: Mosby/Elsevier, pp1948–9.

→ http://emedicine.medscape.com/article/820200-overview

5. B ★★★★ OHEM, 4th edn → pp194–5

This patient's serum paracetamol level is below the normal treatment line but above the high risk treatment line on the paracetamol treatment graph (see Fig. 4.2 on p153). This patient is in high-risk group because of her alcohol consumption and low albumin (she may have cachexia or malnutrition). Alcoholics and patients on hepatic enzyme-inducing drugs such as rifampicin, anticonvulsants, etc. have greater risk of toxicity because of increased production of toxic metabolites of paracetamol. Patients with cachexia, malnutrition, anorexia, cystic fibrosis may have depleted glutathione reserve and be at increased risk of liver damage.

Start treatment with acetylcysteine immediately. There is no indication of giving fresh frozen plasma or haemodialysis.

→ www.toxbase.org/Chemicals/Management-Pages/Paracetamol---adult-management--4h/

6. A ★★★★ OHEM, 4th edn → p204

The patient has moderate alcohol poisoning. The airway is at risk of aspiration. Therefore airway protection and adequate ventilation are the immediate management priorities. As alcohol is rapidly absorbed from the stomach, activated charcoal and gastric lavage are ineffective. Activated charcoal is given orally and it cannot be administered to a patient with GCS score of 8/15. Correct hypoglycaemia by giving 500mL glucose 5% or 250mL 10% IV in such situations, and not glucagon. IV thiamine has no role here as a first-line drug as this patient is unlikely to have alcohol-related thiamine deficiency. In chronic alcoholics, it is important to give the patient thiamine before correcting the hypoglycaemia to avoid precipitation of Wernicke's encephalopathy.

- Mild alcohol poisoning: Serum ethanol level <180mg/dL or 39mmol/L
- Moderate poisoning: Serum ethanol level 180–350mg/dL or 39–76mmol/L
- Severe poisoning: Serum ethanol level 350–450mg/dL or 76–98mmol/L
- Potentially fatal: Serum ethanol level >450mg/dL or >98mmol/L

The serum ethanol level is not routinely measured, but may be requested in such cases. Management of airway or hypoglycaemia does not depend on the serum ethanol levels.

→ www.toxbase.org/Poisons-Index-A-Z/E-Products/
Ethanol--------------/

7. E ★★★★ OHEM, 4th edn → p210

This patient has CO poisoning. This diagnosis is supported by the symptoms the spouse is also having. CO is produced not just by gas but also by the incomplete combustion of all carbon-containing fuels: gas (domestic or bottled), coal, coke, oil, and wood. Stoves, fires and boilers, water heaters, paraffin heaters, and room heaters are all potential sources. Caravans, boats, and mobile homes are also at risk as they often contain portable appliances that use these fuels, and engine or generator exhaust gases can also contain high levels of CO. During incomplete combustion, carbon, hydrogen, and available oxygen combine to form carbon dioxide, water, heat and CO. Any disruption of the burning process or shortage of oxygen can increase CO production and accumulation to dangerous levels.

The immediate management is to remove patient and their cohabitants from the source. Give 100% oxygen by a tightly fitting mask with an inflated face-seal. The patients who remain unconscious may require intubation and ventilation.

Indications for hyperbaric oxygen therapy:

1. The patient has lost consciousness at any stage
2. The patient has neurological signs other than headache
3. Myocardial ischaemia/arrhythmia diagnosed by ECG
4. The patient is pregnant.

This patient may require hyperbaric oxygen therapy, but the immediate management will be oxygen until he is referred for the above therapy. There is no place for non-invasive ventilation. Oxygen is the greater priority than IV fluids.

→ www.toxbase.org/Chemicals/Chemicals/Carbon-monoxide-E/

Extended Matching Questions

1. H ★   OHEM, 4th edn → p190

Heroin is an opioid class of drug with morphine-like actions. It blocks the opioid receptors OP1 (delta), OP2 (kappa), and OP3 (mu), which are distributed through out the central nervous system and peripheral tissues. Stimulation of these receptors by opioids inhibits pain by inhibiting the release of neurotransmitters. In general, opioids cause central nervous system and respiratory depression, and miosis. This patient has self-injected a large dose of heroin IV and developed a respiratory arrest. As heroin is lipophilic, it penetrates the blood–brain barrier rapidly and acts within 1min of IV injection, and 3–5min of intranasal administration. The immediate management is to give IM naloxone 400–800mcg. Later in the ED the patient needs to be given IV naloxone infusion as the half-life of naloxone is very short. Naloxone is the specific competitive antagonist at the opioid receptors.

→ www.toxbase.org/Poisons-Index-A-Z/H-Products/
Heroin----------------------/

2. D ★   OHEM, 4th edn → p198

This elderly patient has received a small dose of morphine but a large dose of midazolam within a very short period of time. Midazolam is a benzodiazepine, which produces sedative, hypnotic, anxiolytic and anticonvulsant effects by enhancing the inhibitory actions of GABA. In overdoses, it produces central nervous system depression. Respiratory depression is seen in large overdoses, particularly when used in combination with opioids.

Flumazenil is the antidote of choice as it is a non-specific, competitive antagonist of the benzodiazepine receptors. The usual initial dose is 200mcg, and may be gradually increased if it is not effective.

Flumazenil should be used carefully as it may precipitate convulsions and arrhythmias. Therefore, careful monitoring is necessary while using this drug and in the UK it is only licensed for in-hospital overdoses.

→ www.toxbase.org/Poisons-Index-A-Z/M-Products/Midazolam/

3. J ★ OHEM, 4th edn → p196

The symptoms are suggestive of tricyclic antidepressant poisoning. The patient's GCS score is 9/15 and she has ECG changes. She is also acidotic (metabolic acidosis). An IV bolus dose of 50–100mL of 8.4% sodium bicarbonate may result in a dramatic improvement in the patient's condition. Sodium bicarbonate alters the protein-binding site and reduces the availability of active free tricyclic drug.

→ www.toxbase.org/Poisons-Index-A-Z/A-Products/
Amitriptyline----------------/

4. F ★ OHEM, 4th edn → p200

The cardioselectivity of atenolol is lost in overdoses. At the β-receptor level, β-blockers competitively inhibit the catecholamines (adrenaline (epinephrine)). Catecholamines increase myocardial contraction (inotropic effect), increase the heart rate (chronotropic effect) and increase cardiac conduction. β-blockers are rapidly absorbed from the GI tract, reaching peak plasma levels within one to 4h. Most common toxic features are bradycardia followed by hypotension and unconsciousness. Immediate management is oxygen, IV fluids and cardiac monitoring. Activated charcoal may be given within the first hour of ingestion but its benefit is not proven. The initial treatment is atropine 0.5mg IV. It may be ineffective in reversing bradycardia and hypotension. The next and the best treatment is glucagon (2–10mg IV), which does not depend on β-receptors for its actions. It has both inotropic and chronotropic actions based on its activation of the myocardial adenylatecyclase system, producing dramatic improvement in pulse, BP, and return of consciousness.

→ www.toxbase.org/Poisons-Index-A-Z/A-Products/
Atenolol-------------/

5. J ★ OHEM, 4th edn → pp194–5

Paracetamol overdose is treated by following a treatment nomogram (Fig. 4.2). The minimum serum paracetamol level requiring treatment is 200mg/L in low-risk patients and 100mg/L in the high-risk group (see SBA Answer 5 and Fig. 4.2 below for details of high-risk group). As the paracetamol level is <200mg/L, this patient does not require treatment with acetylcysteine.

This patient's salicylate level denotes moderate poisoning (mild <450mg/L, moderate >450mg/L and severe >700mg/L). The aims of treatment are to reduce absorption from the GI tract, correct the dehydration and acid–base abnormality, and to increase excretion via the kidneys. Activated charcoal is effective in reducing absorption if given within 1h of ingestion. In mild cases, hydration may be achieved by increasing intake of oral fluids. In moderate poisoning, in addition to IV fluids, patients need sodium bicarbonate infusion 1.26% to alkalize the urine to a pH of 7–8, which increases the rate of salicylate excretion through the kidneys. Severe poisoning may require haemodialysis with other supportive measures.

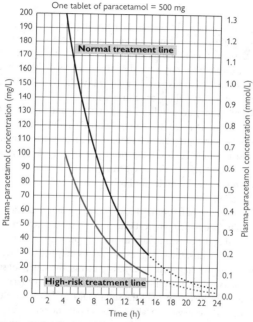

One tablet of paracetamol = 500 mg

Normal treatment line

High-risk treatment line

Plasma-paracetamol concentration (mg/L)

Plasma-paracetamol concentration (mmol/L)

Time (h)

Plasma concentration of paracetamol vs time. Patients whose plasma-paracetamol concentrations are above the **normal treatment line** should be treated with N-acetylcysteine by intravenous infusion (or, provided the overdose has been taken **within 10–12h** with methionine by mouth. See *Paracetmolo poisioning*). Patients on enzyme-including drugs (e.g. carbamazepine, phenobarbital, phenytion, rifampicin, and alcohol) or who are malnourished (e.g. in anorexia, in alcholism, or those who are HIV-positive) should be treated if their plasma-paracetamol concentractions are above the **high-risk treatment line**.

→ www.toxbase.org/Poisons-Index-A-Z/S-Products/Salicylates/

CHAPTER 5

INFECTIOUS DISEASES

'The physician who killed me neither bled, purged or pilled
me, nor counted my pulse, but it comes to the same, in the
height of my fever I thought of his name.'

Nicarchus

An infectious disease, as the name implies, is caused by
pathogenic microorganisms such as bacteria, viruses,
parasites, and fungi, and it spreads from one person to
another through various ways, directly or indirectly. Most, but
not all, of such diseases present to the ED with fever. Septic
shock, respiratory failure, or central nervous system
involvement may occur following an infection and threaten life.
Such a situation presenting with tachycardia, reduced BP,
tachypnoea, or depressed GCS requires immediate assessment
and resuscitation. Following the principles of ABCDE, promptly
carry out airway protection, oxygenation, and IV access with
collection of blood samples for investigations, and fluid
resuscitation.

The aetiology of fever may be wide ranging, but a careful
history and a detailed physical examination should help in
determining the cause in majority of cases presenting to the ED.
In addition to this, the initial investigations may help further in
establishing the diagnosis. In elderly patients, the source of such
infections may be the respiratory system, the genitourinary
system or the involvement of the soft tissues, and they are often
serious. In the otherwise healthy younger patient, one must
keep in mind the other systems such as the central nervous
system, as well as abdominal and soft tissue infections. Patients
may often present in septic shock.

Even if the cause of a fever may not be evident at the outset,
the best 'guestimate' often helps in determining which
antibiotics to start with, which should be given as soon as the
culture samples have been collected. One must make every
effort to collect appropriate samples of body fluids (blood, urine,
stool, sputum, etc.) to find the source of infection so that

targeted antimicrobial therapy may be started if the empirical treatment has not worked. A discussion with the on-call microbiologist to properly direct the empirical antibiotic therapy is often most rewarding.

A patient with an infectious disease may put others at risk as well, resulting in devastating effects, particularly in hospitals. It is also our duty to take care to protect others, besides trying to limit the contagion as much as possible by following some basic principles of handwashing, keeping forearms and hands bare below the elbows, tying hair tidily at the back, refraining from wearing wristwatches, jewellery, etc.—all matters of common sense.

An ED should welcome *all* patients coming through its doors, however, this consequently and potentially also brings in a host of uninvited pathogens. It is extremely important not to forget about MRSA and *Clostridium difficile*. Some patients are known to have MRSA; many others are resistant to commonly used antibiotics, while yet others develop colitis due to hospital-acquired *C. difficile*. This must be kept in the mind while approaching the patient with the first dose of an injection of antibiotics! ■

SINGLE BEST ANSWERS

1. A 18-year-old woman is being brought to the ED by a blue light ambulance in a semiconscious state after suffering from headache, vomiting, fever, and neck stiffness for last couple of days. Her temperature is 38.8°C, heart rate 120bpm, BP 100/70mmHg, and GCS score 10/15, and she has purpuric rash all over her body. Which is the *single* most likely organism responsible? ★

A *Escherichia coli*

B *Haemophilus influenzae*

C *Listeria monocytogenes*

D *Neisseria meningitidis*

E *Streptococcus pneumoniae*

2. A 19-year-old woman from a nearby university is in a semiconscious state after suffering from headache, vomiting, fever, and neck stiffness for the past couple of days. Her temperature is 39.0°C, heart rate 124bpm, BP 106/70mmHg, and GCS score 11/15, and she has purpuric rash all over her body. Which is the *single* most appropriate immediate management? ★

A Ampicillin

B Ceftriaxone

C Chloramphenicol

D Rifampicin

E Vancomycin

3. A 25-year-old woman with soreness around her genitalia had unprotected sex a few days ago. She feels unwell and has developed small groups of multiple lesions with a red base and the surrounding area is sore to touch. The patient's temperature is 37.8°C, and the inguinal lymph nodes are mildly tender. Which is the *single* most likely causative organism? ★

A *Chlamydia trachomatis*

B *Haemophilus ducreyi*

C *Herpes simplex*

D *Treponema pallidum*

E *Varicella zoster*

4. A 35-year-old woman with soreness around her genitalia had unprotected sex a few days ago. She feels unwell and has developed small groups of multiple lesions with a red base and the surrounding area is sore to touch. Her temperature is 37.8°C, and her inguinal lymph nodes are mildly tender. Which is the *single* most appropriate treatment? ★

A Aciclovir

B Azithromycin

C Ceftriaxone

D Combivir

E Doxycycline

5. A 45-year-old man attends the ED with pain and purulent discharge from an abdominal wound. He had a left hemicolectomy for carcinoma of the descending colon 3 weeks ago and MRSA wound infection. Which is the *single* most appropriate measure to avoid spreading of the infection? ★

A Allowing only MRSA-negative staff to take care of him

B Asking the patient to wash his hands frequently

C Cleaning the isolation room frequently with special antiseptics

D Only MRSA-negative relatives should visit him

E Wearing protective equipment during every visit

6. A 55-year-old man attends the ED a week after receiving a laceration on his left thigh following a fall in a park. He is now unwell and in considerable pain. His pulse rate is 128bpm and temperature 39.3°C. The skin surrounding the wound is discoloured and swollen and makes a crackling sound on palpation. The discharge from the wound is serous with a sweet odour. Which is the *single* most likely causative organism? ★

A *Clostridium botulinum*

B *Clostridium histolyticum*

C *Clostridium perfringens*

D *Clostridium septicum*

E *Clostridium tetani*

7. A 78-year-old man has had a band-like pain around his left lower chest for about 3 days. He now has red lesions with some crusting along the left chest wall spreading from his back to the front along the ribs. Which is the *single* most appropriate treatment? ★

A Aciclovir

B Combivir

C Erythromycin

D Flucloxacillin

E Penicillin

8. A 19-year-old man has a sore throat and has had difficulty swallowing for 3 days. He feels unwell, tired, and hot. His temperature is 38°C. His tonsils are enlarged and have red with white spots on the surface. The lymph nodes in the neck are tender. The white cell count is 11.5×10^9/L, neutrophils 5.6×10^9/L, lymphocytes 7.2×10^9/L with a few atypical cells, monocytes 0.8×10^9/L and platelets 300×10^9/L. Which is the *single* most likely causative organism? ★

A Cytomegalovirus

B Epstein–Barr virus

C Group B β-haemolytic streptococcus

D HSV

E *Toxoplasma gondii*

9. A 22-year-old woman attends the ED asking for an HIV test. A condom had split when she was having intercourse the night before with an unknown person from sub-Saharan Africa. Which is the *single* most appropriate management? ★

A Asking her to return after 3 months for testing

B Reassuring her that the possibility of infection is negligible

C Referral to GP for follow-up

D Referral to the next genitourinary clinic

E Taking a blood sample for testing for HIV

10. A 19-year-old woman has attended the ED asking for an HIV test. After a visit to a nightclub the day before, she had unprotected intercourse with an unknown man from sub-Saharan Africa. Which is the *single* most important mode of transmission of HIV infection from the man? ★

A Alveolar fluid

B Salivary secretions

C Semen

D Sweat

E Vaginal fluid

11. A 42-year-old man has been coughing with yellow expectoration, feeling of hot and cold with sweats, and worsening shortness of breath for 4–5 days. He is HIV positive and an IV drug user. His temperature is 38.3°C, heart rate 112bpm, and respiratory rate 28breaths/min. His chest X-ray shows consolidation in the right mid zone. Which is the *single* most likely diagnosis? ★

A Cytomegaloviral pneumonia

B *Haemophilus influenzae* pneumonia

C *Pneumocystis jiroveci* pneumonia

D Pulmonary tuberculosis

E Streptococcal pneumonia

12. A 25-year-old woman has become unwell with a headache, vomiting, and fever. She has injected heroin several times in the past. At the site of the most recent injection she has redness, pain, and haemorrhagic blisters and there is tenderness surrounding the area of the injection. Her temperature is 38.8°C, heart rate 120bpm, and BP 100/70mmHg. Which is the *single* most likely causative organism? ★ ★

A *Bacteroides fragilis*

B *Clostridium perfringens*

C *Klebsiella* sp.

D *Pseudomonas aeruginosa*

E *Streptococcus pyogenes*

13. A 34-year-old man has had headaches, body aches, and fever with rigors and severe sweating for 2 days. He has recently returned from the Gambia where he was working for a charity organization. He has taken several medications, including antimalarials. His heart rate is 110bpm and temperature 37.5 °C. Which is the *single* most important immediate diagnostic test? ★ ★

A Blood culture

B Chest X-ray

C Liver function tests

D Peripheral blood film

E Urine culture

14. A 42-year-old man has had headaches, body aches, and fever with rigors and severe sweating for 2 days. He recently returned from Guinea, where he was working for a charity organization. He has taken several medications, including antimalarial tablets. His temperature is 37.5°C and heart rate 110bpm. Which is the *single* most likely causative organism? ★ ★

A *Plasmodium bubalis*

B *Plasmodium falciparum*

C *Plasmodium malariae*

D *Plasmodium ovale*

E *Plasmodium vivax*

ANSWERS

Single Best Answers

1. D ★

Neisseria meningitidis is the predominant organism in children below the age of 5 years and young adults between the ages of 14 and 24 years. Five major serogroups cause most of the meningococcal disease worldwide (A, B, C, Y, and W-135). In 2008–9, 1166 cases of meningococcal disease were reported in the UK, out of which 1052 and 13 cases were caused by serogroups B and C respectively. Serogroup A meningitis is rare in the UK but has caused large numbers of deaths in other parts of the world such as sub-Saharan Africa.

A: In the UK, most cases of *Escherichia coli* meningitis occur in newborn babies. It can also occur in those with suppressed immune systems weakened by AIDS, cancer, diabetes and other disorders, plus use of some immunosuppressants. It can also be as a result of a head injury or surgery to the head, which allows the bacteria to enter. CSF shunts (which are used to drain excess fluid from around the brain to relieve pressure) can also allow this to happen.

B: Hib is common in babies and children below the age of 4 years. A conjugate vaccine to protect against Hib was introduced in 1992 to protect young children and is now offered to all children at 2, 3, and 4 months of age with a booster at 12 months. Before this, 1 in 600 children contracted Hib before the age of 5 years, and it was responsible for about 70 deaths and 150 cases of brain damage a year. Because of the success of the vaccine, Hib meningitis in now rare and cases of Hib meningitis have reduced by over 90% in the UK.

C: *Listeria* meningitis is caused when the infection invades the nervous system. It occurs mainly in babies, elderly people, and those with weakened immune systems. It can be passed from mother to baby during pregnancy or while giving birth. Meningitis mainly occurs in babies who get ill 2–3 days after birth, with the most common complications being pneumonia and respiratory distress. The infection is uncommon in the UK largely due to successful education campaigns about the dangers of eating unpasteurized milk products or contaminated poultry or shellfish.

E: Group B streptococcus, also known as GBS or group B strep, is the most common cause of severe infection in newborn babies in the UK. Pregnant women can transmit GBS to their newborns at birth. The disease in newborns usually occurs in the first week of life—known as 'early-onset'. Babies can also get a slightly less serious 'late-onset' form that develops a week to a few months after birth. In the UK, about 340 babies a year develop a GBS infection. Babies who survive can be left with speech, hearing, and vision problems as well as learning disabilities.

→ www.meningitisuk.org/about-meningitis/bacterial-meningitis.htm

→ www.hpa.org.uk/web/HPAweb&HPAwebStandard/ HPAweb_C/1234859711901?printable=true

2. B ★   OHEM, 4th edn →pp228–9

The first-line antibiotic in suspected cases of meningococcal septicaemia is cefotaxime or ceftriaxone IV, the 'third generation' cephalosporins. They are indicated in septicaemia, pneumonia, and meningitis (excellent coverage for *Streptococcus pneumoniae* and *Haemophilus influenzae*).

A: Ampicillin, a broad-spectrum penicillin, is active against certain Gram-positive and Gram-negative organisms but is inactivated by penicillinases, including those produced by *Staphylococcus aureus* and by common Gram-negative bacilli such as *Escherichia coli*. Almost 60% of *E. coli* and 20% of *H. influenzae* strains are now resistant. Ampicillin and gentamicin are used jointly in *Listeria* meningitis to cover *Listeria* infections in individuals >55 years. Give vancomycin ± rifampicin if the organism is suspected to be penicillin-resistant pneumococcus.

C: Chloramphenicol may be given to patients with a history of immediate hypersensitivity to penicillin or cephalosporins after consulting with a microbiologist.

D: Rifampicin is used as secondary prophylaxis in the dose of 600mg every 12h for 2 days. The other drugs used in such prophylaxis are ciprofloxacin 500mg as a single dose or ceftriaxone (unlicensed indication) 250mg IM as a single dose.

E: Vancomycin, a glycopeptide antibiotic has bactericidal activity against aerobic and anaerobic Gram-positive bacteria including multiresistant staphylococci. It is used IV in the treatment of endocarditis and other serious infections caused by Gram-positive cocci. Oral preparations are effective in the treatment of *Clostridium difficile* infection. Vancomycin may be used in combination with third-generation cephalosporins or rifampicin if the organism is suspected to be penicillin-resistant pneumococcus.

For more information, see *BNF* 59, March 2010, section 5.1.

3. C ★   OHEM, 4th edn →pp243–5

The patient has characteristic signs of genital herpes infection caused by HSV. HSV type 2 (HSV-2) is the commonest offending organism, but genital lesions may also be caused by HSV-1. Patients usually develop symptoms between 2 and 7 days after the exposure. Sexually transmitted diseases may be broadly divided into two categories: ulcerative and non-ulcerative.

- Examples of ulcerative diseases: herpes, primary syphilis, chancroid, Lymphogranuloma venereum, pyoderma, trauma, etc.
- Examples of non-ulcerative diseases: chlamydia, gonorrhoea, secondary/tertiary syphilis, *Candida*, etc.

Chlamydia trachomatis not only causes chlamydia but certain specific serotypes are also responsible for lymphogranuloma venereum. The genital lesions are small and painless, followed by inguinal lymphadenopathy and development of sinuses.

Haemophilus ducreyi causes chancroid, which is common in developing countries. About a week after the exposure, the patient develops a small, red, tender papule, which breaks down to form multiple shallow painful ulcers and inguinal lymphadenopathy. Sometimes it may be difficult to distinguish from herpes.

Treponema pallidum causes syphilis, the ulcers of which are painless. The ulcers have a smooth, slightly raised edge, with sharply defined borders and a clean base.

Varicella zoster is responsible for chicken pox and shingles. The distribution of shingles is along the dermatomes, mostly in the thoracic region.

4. A ★   OHEM, 4th edn →pp243–5

The patient has characteristic signs of genital herpes infection caused by HSV. HSV type 2 (HSV-2) is the commonest offending organism, but genital lesions may also be caused by HSV-1. Patients usually develop symptoms between 2 and 7 days after the exposure. Aciclovir in primary genital herpes reduces shedding of the viral load, thereby reducing the transmission. It also reduces the frequency of recurrence of the disease.

Combivir is a combination of antiviral drugs (zidovudine and lamivudine) used in the treatment of HIV infections.

Infectious diseases

Azithromycin is used in treatment of chancroid and chlamydia, which is also treated by doxycycline. Doxycycline is also the drug of choice in lymphogranuloma venereum. Ceftriaxone may be used for the treatment of gonorrhoea and chancroid (second-line drug).

→ www.cdc.gov/std/treatment/2006/genital-ulcers.htm

5. E ★   OHEM, 4th edn →p240

MRSA is a bacterium that causes infections which are difficult to treat as it is resistant to many antibiotics. MRSA is a commensal on the skin or in the nose of 20–40% of people. Transmission is minimized by handwashing and other infection control measures as mentioned in the following URLs. As a result of infection control measures the incidence of hospital-acquired MRSA is under constant decline as shown by the Health Protection Agency.

→ www.hpa.org.uk/web/HPAwebFile/HPAweb_C/1194947417699

→ www.hpa.org.uk/web/HPAwebFile/HPAweb_C/1194947365238

→ www.hpa.org.uk/webw/HPAweb&HPAwebStandard/
HPAweb_C/1237448960576?p=1158945065017

6. C ★   OHEM, 4th edn →p242

The patient has a highly lethal gas gangrene infection, which is caused by the exotoxin-producing Gram-positive anaerobic clostridia. *Clostridium perfringens* is responsible for 80–90% of the infections. *Clostridium septicum* and *Clostridium histolyticum* cause only 10–20% cases. *Clostridium tetani* causes tetanus and *Clostridium botulinum* causes botulism by producing a toxin in food.

Gas gangrene is a rapidly spreading infection of muscle. It may involve wounds of the buttocks, amputations related to vascular disease, or severe muscle injuries. The patient develops sudden and severe pain at the site of the wound with generalized toxicity (tachycardia, fever, and sweating). A serous discharge from the wound, with surrounding skin discolouration and locally present haemorrhagic vesicles and swelling. The site may be very tender with crepitus. The patient requires urgent surgical treatment to remove all infected tissues, antibiotics (metronidazole with penicillin or clindamycin), and possibly hyperbaric oxygen therapy and gas gangrene antitoxin.

7. A ★   OHEM, 4th edn →p245

The patient has shingles, which is generally distributed along a dermatome. It commonly involves the thorax but it can also involve the face (geniculate ganglion) or eyes and other areas. It starts with a band-like burning pain and hypersensitivity of the skin followed by erythema and vesicle formation 1–4 days after the onset of pain.

These then form crusts and heal in about 3–4 weeks. Shingles occurs in people who have contracted chicken pox in the past. The herpes zoster virus remains dormant in the dorsal root ganglion and erupts as shingles if the immunity of the host is compromised.

Shingles should be treated with aciclovir, famciclovir, or valaciclovir, which reduces post-herpetic pain if given early. Antibiotics may be needed if the patient has secondary infection. Patients usually also require analgesia.

Combivir is a combination of the antiviral drugs used in the treatment of HIV infection.

8. B ★ OHEM, 4th edn → p246

The patient has glandular fever caused by Epstein–Barr virus or human herpes virus-4. This condition classically affects school children and college students (young adults). The infection spreads via droplets while kissing. This acute viral syndrome is characterized by fever, exudative pharyngotonsillitis, cervical lymphadenopathy, and peripheral lymphocytosis with atypical lymphocytes. This patient has all these features. In severe cases the tonsillar swelling may cause breathing difficulty. The finding of a lymphocytosis >50% or raised antibodies (Monospot) suggest the diagnosis. The antibodies are sensitive and specific, but may be negative initially. Differential diagnoses include CMV infection and toxoplasmosis (*Toxoplasma gondii*). Glandular fever generally resolves in 1–3 weeks. In severe infections a high dose of steroids may be given. An antibiotic is indicated only if the patient is suspected to have a concurrent streptococcal infection. The Monospot test may help in distinguishing infectious mononucleosis from CMV infection and toxoplasmosis. The Monospot test detects heterophil antibodies, which develop in 90% of patients by week 3, disappearing after about 3 months. In the 10% of cases in which the Monospot test is negative, especially in the early stages of the disease, the diagnosis may be confirmed by detecting EBM-specific IgM antibodies in the blood. Peripheral blood smears demonstrate atypical mononuclear cells in 75% of patients, which may also be present in viral infections such as CMV, HIV, etc. and toxoplasmosis, lymphoma, leukaemia, etc.

A: Most healthy children and adults infected with CMV have no symptoms and may not even know that they have been infected. Others may develop a mild illness. Symptoms include fever, sore throat, fatigue, and swollen glands. In adults, the infection may be severe in immunocompromised or elderly patients.

C: In group B β-haemolytic streptococcus infection the neutrophil count would be expected to be raised as opposed to lymphocytosis.

D: HSV may cause pharyngitis, affecting typically young adults, and can be due to primary infection or reactivation. It is characterized by the presence of painful vesicles with erythematous bases associated with ulcers on the pharynx, lips, tongue, etc.

E: Toxoplasmosis is caused by the parasite *T. gondii* and may cause symptoms similar to glandular fever. Most healthy adults do not have any symptoms or experience minimal flu-like symptoms. The symptoms of headache, confusion, fever, sore throat may be severe in immunocompromised patients.

For additional information, see the *Oxford Handbook of Clinical Medicine*, 8th edn, p401.

9. D ★   OHEM, 4th edn →p248

The patient should be referred to the local genitourinary clinic for further advice on HIV testing and counselling. She may be given PEP in the ED as soon as possible, which is continued for 1 month. As the patient had had sex with someone from a high prevalence area, the chances of getting HIV infection may be considerable. For information on indications for PEP, see: http://www.bashh.org/documents/58/58.pdf

HIV infection is detected by presence of antibodies, which may not appear until 3 months after exposure. HIV testing is not an appropriate investigation for the ED. The testing should be done in special clinics where facilities for informed consent and counselling are available.

→ www.parliament.uk/documents/upload/postpn297.pdf

→ www.avert.org/uk-statistics.htm

→ http://hcd2.bupa.co.uk/fact_sheets/html/aids.html

10. C ★   OHEM, 4th edn →p248

HIV has been isolated from variety of body fluids: blood and blood products, serum, semen, vaginal secretions, urine, CSF, tears, breast milk, alveolar fluid, synovial fluid, bone marrow, and saliva. Only a few modes of transmission have been established: unscreened blood/blood products (blood transfusion before 1985 in the UK), semen, vaginal secretions, breast milk and transplacental.

→ www.parliament.uk/documents/upload/postpn297.pdf

→ www.avert.org/uk-statistics.htm

→ http://hcd2.bupa.co.uk/fact_sheets/html/aids.html

11. E ★ OHEM, 4th edn →p250

Patients with productive cough and fever with focal consolidation on chest X-ray are likely to have bacterial pneumonia. IV drug abusers are at special risk of bacterial infections such as streptococcal pneumonia or *Haemophilus influenzae* infections.

A and C: CMV or *Pneumocystis jiroveci* (previously *Pneumocystis carinii*) or pneumonia (PCP) is more likely if the patient has a dry cough with evidence of diffuse bilateral interstitial infiltration on chest X-ray.

B: *Haemophilus influenzae* is the second commonest cause of pneumonia in such situations.

D: The incidence of pulmonary tuberculosis in HIV-infected patients has increased recently. The main presenting symptoms and signs are cough, fever, and haemoptysis. The chest X-ray may show cavitations in upper zone with hilar lymphadenopathy.

→ www.avert.org/hiv-opportunistic-infections.htm

12. E ★ ★ OHEM, 4th edn →p239

The patient is developing necrotizing fasciitis at the site of the injection. This is a rare but severe, bacterial soft tissue infection. The most commonly implicated organism is *Streptococcus pyogenes*. But other organisms may also be involved, e.g. *Staphylococcus aureus*, *Bacteroides*, clostridia, etc. Treatment involves resuscitation with IV fluids, antibiotics, and surgery to debride the affected area.

13. D ★ ★ OHEM, 4th edn →p253

The patient has returned from sub-Saharan Africa, where *Plasmodium falciparum* malaria is prevalent. Malaria often develops despite antimalarial treatment because of drug resistance or incorrect dosage. Ask for the report on the peripheral blood film to be ready within 1h. Blood and urine culture reports will take a few days. Chest X-ray and liver function tests are important to assess or exclude other diagnoses and risks, respectively.

→ http://www.britishinfection.org/drupal/sites/default/files/malariatreatmentBIS07.pdf

14. B ★ ★ OHEM, 4th edn →p253

The patient has returned from sub-Saharan Africa, where *Plasmodium falciparum* malaria is prevalent. *P. falciparum* also occurs in travellers from South-East Asia, and Central and South America. Other variants of malarial parasites are prevalent in different parts of the world, e.g. *Plasmodium vivax* in South Asia and *Plasmodium bubalis* infects apes, lemurs (not humans).

P. falciparum produces fulminating disease, with severe organ damage and subsequently death. Its incubation period is 7–10 days and symptoms recur at 36–48h; 90% of patients present within 1 month with a flu-like prodrome: headache, malaise, myalgia, and anorexia, followed by fever paroxysms as above. Patients may have anaemia, jaundice, or hepatosplenomegaly. Peripheral blood films (both thick and thin) may show sausage-shaped gametocytes in RBC ghosts.

Plasmodium vivax and *Plasmodium ovale* infections have an incubation period of 10–17 days and the fever spikes every 48h. Both may produce true relapses by new invasion of the blood from latent hypnozoites in the liver up to a few years after complete clearance of parasites from the blood. *P. vivax* malaria is also called 'benign tertian malaria'.

Plasmodium malariae has an incubation period of 18–40 days. The fever peaks every 72h (quartan malaria). It is rarely fatal but may cause glomerulonephritis.

For additional information, see the *Oxford Handbook of Clinical Medicine*, 8th edn, pp394–5.

→ http://www.britishinfection.org/drupal/sites/default/files/ MalariaAlgorithm07.pdf

→ www.cdc.gov/malaria/distribution_epi/epidemiology.htm

CHAPTER 6

ENVIRONMENTAL EMERGENCIES

'Cold! If the thermometer had been an inch longer we'd have frozen to death.'

Mark Twain

Environmental emergencies comprise acute exposure of human beings to extremes of temperature, electrical, and radiation injuries, drowning and diving, and high-altitude sickness. Of these, hypothermia, electrical injuries, and drowning are slightly more commonly encountered. However, there are some parts of the UK where scuba diving incidents are more frequent.

The story of a physician surviving a temperature of 13.7°C after a 9h resuscitation effort, or various war tragedies in which thousands of soldiers died during cold exposure, etc., are well known. Hypothermia occurs when the core body temperature drops below 35°C, and the compensatory mechanism in a healthy individual is overwhelmed by the extreme exposure. This may be sometimes hastened by various types of medications affecting the thermoregulation.

The management in the ED starts with basics (ABCDE). While the ABC and D are taken care of, an accurate measurement of temperature is essential, and most EDs do so by measuring an oesophageal, rectal, or bladder temperature, while the patient is being warmed. The common rhythm in a cardiac arrest associated with hypothermia is asystole. But if the patient is in VF, defibrillation is usually unsuccessful until the core temperature is well above 28–30°C. Therefore, rewarming continues alongside resuscitation and as the core temperature rises, defibrillation attempts should continue according to the UK resuscitation guidelines.

The approximate death rate from drowning in the UK is 0.72/100 000 population per year. In 2005, of 435 deaths from drowning, 39 cases were between the ages of 0 and 14 years.

Alcohol consumption in the vicinity of water is a major risk factor for morbidity or death by drowning. During the initial assessment, important details surrounding the incident should be obtained rapidly. The outcome of patients in cardiac arrest, who are often hypothermic as well, largely depends on how quickly CPR is initiated. The duration of CPR remains controversial in the hypothermic drowned patient—a safe approach is to continue until the core temperature reaches 35°C.

This chapter includes questions on hypothermia, drowning, and some other environmental emergencies to give the reader an insight into the latest management of these situations. ■

SINGLE BEST ANSWERS

1. A 78-year-old woman has been brought in by a blue light ambulance after being found on the floor by her neighbours. She opens her eyes to voice, makes confused conversations and withdraws on painful stimulus. Her temperature is 32°C, heart rate is 60bpm, BP 100/60mmHg, respiratory rate 12breaths/min, and capillary blood glucose 4.2mmol/L. Which is the *single* most appropriate immediate management? ★

A Arranging endotracheal intubation

B Giving 50mL of 50% glucose

C Giving 400µg of naloxone

D Giving 2L of normal saline

E Wrapping her up with warm blankets

2. A 22-year-old woman has been brought in by a blue light ambulance after being found on the roadside in a hit-and-run incident. She has a swollen right thigh. Her temperature is 31°C, heart rate 60bpm, BP 100/60mmHg, and respiratory rate 12breaths/min. She is confused. Which is the *single* most appropriate method of rewarming her? ★

A Heat pads

B Hot air blanket

C Hot water bottles

D Space blankets

E Warm water bath

3. A 75-year-old woman has been brought in by a blue light ambulance after being found on the floor by her neighbours. Her temperature is 33°C, heart rate 60bpm, BP 100/60mmHg, respiratory rate 12breaths/min, and bedside capillary blood glucose 4.0mmol/L. She has been covered with warm blankets and given warm humidified oxygen. Which is the *single* most appropriate explanation of the way the blankets would help in rewarming her? ★

A The autonomic nervous system is suppressed

B Dissipation of heat is minimized

C The endocrine system is activated

D Exogenous heat is transferred to the patient

E Thermal perception is increased

4. A 30-year-old man has been found lying face down in a village stream. He had been seen in a pub a few hours earlier drinking 15 pints of lager in a competition with a friend. His heart rate is 90bpm, BP 100/60mmHg, and respiratory rate 8breaths/min with noisy breathing. He opens his eyes to pain, withdraws on application of a painful stimulus, and is uttering incomprehensible sounds. Which is the *single* most appropriate immediate step of airway management? ★

A Bag valve ventilation

B Endotracheal intubation

C Non-rebreathing mask

D Oropharyngeal airway insertion

E Upper airway suction

5. An 82-year-old man has a headache and fatigue, nausea, severe sweating, dizziness, and weakness after walking to the corner shop on a hot day. His temperature is 39.5°C, heart rate 100bpm, BP 140/82mmHg (lying), and 105/80mmHg (standing). Which is the *single* most important immediate management? ★

A Giving 1g oral paracetamol

B Giving 1L of hypotonic saline solution over 8h

C Giving 2L of normal saline rapidly

D Giving IV dantrolene

E Removing the clothes with cooling by fan

6. A 68-year-old man has been found lying face down in a village stream. He had been seen in a pub a few hours earlier drinking 15 pints of lager in a competition with a friend. His temperature is 31°C, heart rate 90bpm, BP 100/60mmHg, and respiratory rate 4breaths/min with noisy breathing. He opens his eyes to pain, withdraws on application of a painful stimulus and is uttering incomprehensible sounds. Which is the *single* most important good prognostic factor in this patient? ★ ★

A Age

B Alcohol consumption

C Body temperature

D Level of consciousness

E Submersion time

7. A 22-year-old man has pain in both his shoulders and elbows, a headache, generalized erythema, nausea, and vertigo following a sea dive earlier in the day. Which is the *single* most important immediate management? ★ ★

A Chlorphenamine maleate

B Entonox

C Ibuprofen

D Oxygen

E Prochlorperazine

8. A 45-year-old man has lost his way while walking back home in icy weather. He has pain in his feet. After removal of his tight boots his toes are grey and white in colour and feel hard and cold. He has a couple of small blisters. Which is the *single* most appropriate management? ★ ★ ★ ★

A Puncturing the blisters

B Rapidly warming the feet by applying strong heat (45–50°C)

C Warming his toes by gentle rubbing

D Warming the feet in water (35–36°C)

E Warming the feet in water (37–39°C)

9. Four men aged between 25 and 35 have red, burning, and profusely watering eyes, coughing, and a sensation of tightness in the chest after a suspected gas leakage at the factory in which they were working. They also have some redness and irritation of their skin all over the body. They are talking in full sentences. Which is the *single* most important immediate management option? ★ ★ ★ ★

A Arranging an antidote

B Arranging chest X-rays

C Arranging decontamination

D Giving salbutamol nebulizers

E Performing arterial blood gases

ANSWERS

Single Best Answers

1. E ★   OHEM, 4th edn → pp260–2

The patient is mildly hypothermic (mild hypothermia 32–35°C, moderate hypothermia 30–32°C and severe hypothermia <30°C). The primary management is gradual passive rewarming to start with to raise the temperature at a rate of 0.6°C/h particularly in elderly people to prevent hypotension; otherwise cerebral/pulmonary oedema may develop. In adults, the rate of rewarming should be between 0.5°C and 2°C/h. The patient does not require endotracheal intubation as her GCS score is 11 (E3, V4, M4). She should be given warm humidified oxygen via a mask. There is no indication to give naloxone. The respiratory rate is depressed because of hypothermia.

50% glucose is indicated when the finger prick glucose level drops below 4.0mmol/L. Such reading may be falsely low, so re-measure the level after slight rewarming. Generally IV fluid is not required. If the BP drops during rewarming, give 300–500mL of warm 0.9% saline or colloid. Unstable patients should have central venous pressure monitoring and urinary catheter.

2. B ★   OHEM, 4th edn → pp260–2

The patient is moderately hypothermic (see above). The primary management is gradual passive rewarming to start with to raise the temperature at a rate of 0.5–2°C/h. A hot air blanket (The Bair Hugger®) is convenient and often helpful, mainly by reducing heat loss. It circulates hot air through a blanket. The air exits from apertures on the patient's side of the cover, which allows a convective transfer of heat.

Heat pads or hot water bottles are less efficient and can cause burns. Space blankets should be avoided as they are noisy and have no advantage over polythene sheets. A water bath at 37–41°C is rapid and useful for acute immersion hypothermia, but cannot be used in injured patients or if CPR is required.

3. B ★ OHEM, 4th edn → pp260–3

The normal process of heat dissipation is minimized by passive external rewarming. Normal heat loss occurs through five mechanisms:

- 55–65% through radiation
- 2–3% through conduction, which may increase up to five times in wet clothing and up to 25 times in cold water
- 10–12% through convection, which increases with shivering
- 2–9% through respiration
- 20–27% through evaporation from lungs and skin.

Following passive external rewarming by blankets, the heat loss is minimized by reduction of convection, evaporation, and radiation.

A: The serum norepinephrine and epinephrine levels in primates are elevated when the body temperature is reduced from 33°C to 29°C and on rewarming.

Chernow B, Lake CR, Zaritsky A, Finton CK, Casey L, Rainey TG, *et al.* (1983) Sympathetic nervous system 'switch off' with severe hypothermia. *Crit Care Med* **11**(9):677–80.

C: The heat production is decreased in endocrine failure such as myxoedema, hypopituarism, and hypoadrenalism. If a patient fails to rewarm, take a history to find out about any pre-existing endocrine disorder. If this is present, the patient may require hormonal therapy depending on the type of endocrine failure (e.g. for adrenocortical insufficiency administer hydrocortisone, thyroid hormone replacement in myxoedema, etc.)

D: Exogenous heat is transferred in active rewarming performed in cases of severe hypothermia. Active rewarming involves giving patients heated, humidified oxygen, gastric and/or urinary bladder irrigation with warm fluid, peritoneal dialysis using warm peritoneal fluid, etc.

E: External rewarming does not alter the thermal perception, which is reduced in elderly people (inability to sense cold).

Danzi DF (2010) Accidental hypothermia. In: Marx JA, *et al.* (eds) *Rosen's Emergency Medicine: Concepts and Clinical Practice*, 7th edn. Philadelphia: Mosby/Elsevier, pp1868–81.

4. E ★ OHEM, 4th edn → pp266–7

The patient has probably experienced morbidity following drowning after falling in the stream under the influence of alcohol. His GCS score is 8 (E2, V4, M2). The noisy breathing is an indication of water in the respiratory tract. He needs immediate suctioning of his upper airway. Without prior suctioning none of the other airway management options will be successful.

In the past, drowning referred to death within 24h of suffocation from submersion in a liquid, whereas near-drowning was defined as the person surviving at least 24h after the incident regardless of the outcome. The WHO in 2005 defined drowning as 'the process of experiencing respiratory impairment from submersion/immersion in liquid'. The WHO also states that 'drowning outcomes should be classified as: death, morbidity and no morbidity … the terms wet, dry, active, passive, silent, and secondary drowning should no longer be used'. The term 'near-drowning' should not be used.

In adults the commonest predisposing factor is alcohol, sometimes with other drugs. Significant aspiration of fluid into the lungs causes pulmonary vasoconstriction and hypertension with ventilation/perfusion mismatch, aggravated by surfactant destruction and washout, reduced lung compliance, and atelectasis. Acute respiratory failure is common. Arterial blood gas testing shows hypoxia, hypercapnia, and mixed respiratory/metabolic acidosis.

Richards DB, Knaut AL (2010) Drowning. In: Danzi DF (2010) Accidental hypothermia. In: Marx JA, *et al.* (eds) *Rosen's Emergency Medicine: Concepts and Clinical Practice*, 7th edn. Philadelphia: Mosby/Elsevier, p1929.

Van Beeck EF, Branche CM, Sypilman D, Modell JH, Bierens JJLM (2005) A new definition of drowning: Towards documentation and prevention of a global public health problem. *Bull World Health Organ* 83:853.

5. E ★   OHEM, 4th edn → p272

The patient has heat illness, which has a spectrum of severity: heat cramps > heat exhaustion > heat stroke. In heat cramps/exhaustion, homeostatic mechanisms still function, but are overwhelmed. In heat stroke, all thermoregulatory control is lost and body temperature increases rapidly to very high levels (>41°C), causing widespread severe tissue damage and organ damage. In heat cramps the core temperature is between 37°C and 39°C. Core temperature is <40°C in heat exhaustion and >41°C in heat stroke. This patient has features of heat exhaustion.

There is no role for dantrolene or hypotonic solution in this situation. The primary treatment is removal of clothes and cooling by fan. The patient should initially be given oral rehydration fluids. IV fluids should be given cautiously in elderly patients to avoid development of pulmonary or cerebral oedema. Do not give antipyretics.

6. C ★ ★   OHEM, 4th edn → p267

Good prognostic factors:

- Patients who are alert on admission
- Hypothermia
- Older children/adults
- Brief submersion time
- Patients who received rapid basic life support and respond to early resuscitation measures (<10min).

Poor prognostic factors:

- Extremes of age
- Severe acidosis
- Immersion >5min
- Coma on admission.

The patient experienced drowning probably after falling in the stream under the influence of alcohol. His GCS score is 8 (E2, V2, M4). The noisy breathing is an indication of water in the respiratory tract. The good prognostic sign in this patient is hypothermia and presence of vital signs. The poor prognostic signs are age, reduced conscious level, and probably long submersion time (which is unknown). Alcohol is one of the commonest predisposing factors for drowning.

7. D ★ ★   OHEM, 4th edn → pp268–71

The patient probably has DCS. Any symptomatic medication is contraindicated in such a situation, particularly Entonox and anti-inflammatory drugs. Continue to give oxygen 100% until you can discuss the case with a diving physician. There are two types of DCS:

- Type 1 DCS can occur when gas bubbles affect the tissues around skeletal joints. Symptoms usually include unilateral discomfort or pain in one or more joints. The areas most often affected are the knees, elbows, and shoulders. DCS may also present as a cutaneous disorder. Nitrogen bubbles can cause mottling, lumps, or a rash. 'Skin bends', as they are colloquially termed, are more common during hyperbaric chamber 'dives' and when diving using a dry suit. Although not usually in themselves serious, skin symptoms may indicate the presence of problems elsewhere. A particularly serious cutaneous sign of DCS is 'cutis marmorata' marbling, in which an area of skin becomes pale with dark mottling. This is associated with considerable development of inert gas bubbles within the body. If left untreated, type 1 DCS may progress to type 2 DCS.

- Type 2 DCS reflects involvement of the central nervous system and/or the cardiorespiratory system. More than half of those diagnosed with DCS will be classified as type 2. Cerebral symptoms arise from interruption of the blood supply to the main part of the brain, and include confusion, reduced mental function and unconsciousness. Involvement of the cerebellum may lead to tremors, loss of balance ('staggers'), and a lack of coordination (ataxia). Balance may also be affected by damage to the vestibular part of the inner ear. Spinal DCS may present as back pain, paraesthesia, paralysis, and loss of urinary sphincter control—resulting in either incontinence or retention. As discussed already, the formation of small inert gas bubbles does not necessarily lead to the development of DCS. Likewise, when bubbles become trapped in the tiny blood vessels around the lungs' alveoli, problems do not always arise. In fact, it is thought that their accumulation in this area may increase the rate at which the gas is excreted from the body (Edmonds C, Lowry C, Pennefather J (1991)*Diving and Subaquatic Medicine*, 3rd edn, Oxford: Butterworth Heinemann). However, if too many bubbles collect, breathing will become adversely affected ('chokes'). Symptoms include breathlessness, tachypnoea, chest pain, and coughing. Although the symptoms may resolve, this should be regarded as a life-threatening condition as it may progress to fatal respiratory collapse.

→ www.sdm.scot.nhs.uk/decompression_illness/index.htm

→ www.ddrc.org/content/view/88/48/

8. E ★★★★ OHEM, 4th edn → p264

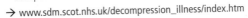

The patient has frostbite of his toes. After exclusion of general body hypothermia and its management, the toes to be treated by immersing the feet in warm water at a temperature of 37–39°C. Once rewarming is started blisters may form; do not puncture them and protect them from injury. Pain after rewarming usually indicates that viable tissue has been successfully rewarmed. Take the following precautions:

- Do not rub the frozen part
- Do not allow the patient to have alcohol or tobacco
- Do not apply ice
- Do not attempt to thaw the frostbitten part in cold water
- Do not attempt to thaw the frostbitten part by using high temperatures, such as those generated by stoves, exhausts, etc.
- Do not break the blisters.

→ www.chems.alaska.gov/EMS/documents/AKColdInj2005.pdf

9. C ★ ★ ★ ★ OHEM, 4th edn → pp264–5

It appears that the men have been exposed to chlorine or phosgene gas after an industrial incident. They have features of inhalation, and eye and skin exposure. The initial steps in their management would include informing seniors, arranging decontamination, and using personal protective equipment before starting treatment as they do not have any life-threatening symptoms or signs. The skin and eyes should be thoroughly washed after removal of their clothes followed by giving oxygen and bronchodilators if necessary. In every ED there will be a CBRN plan and a direct telephone number to call the HPA helpline for advice following such exposures.

→ www.hpa.org.uk/web/HPAwebFile/HPAweb_C/1194947382859

Environmental emergencies

CHAPTER 7
ANALGESIA AND ANAESTHESIA

'Pain is such an uncomfortable feeling that even a tiny amount
of it is enough to ruin every enjoyment.'

Will Rogers

Seventy per cent of patients who present to the ED have
pain as their main complaint—and most of the time as a
sign of injury or inflammation. Therefore, early
assessment by scoring at the point of triage and offering the
appropriate analgesia are the first steps towards the
management of such patients. The College of Emergency
Medicine guidelines suggest that at least 98% of patients in
severe pain (pain score of 7–10) should be offered appropriate
analgesia within 60min of arrival, or triage, whichever is earlier.
In 90% of these patients, the status of pain should be
re-evaluated within 60min of receiving the first dose of the
analgesic. Despite this clear-cut standard and the availability of
a wide variety of analgesics, achieving such a target remains,
occasionally, elusive. It must also be realized that a positive
experience for the patient largely depends on relief of pain as
early as possible. Consequently, one of the primary areas for a
new FY1 to focus on is the pain management. Remember it is
simple and straightforward in most circumstances.

GA may be required in the ED for various clinical indications,
for example, cardioversion, facial trauma or burns, and acute
respiratory failure (such as in asthma). In an emergency
situation it may be a challenging procedure even for an
experienced anaesthetist and could be dangerous for the
patients. An FY1/2 will never be expected to perform this, but it
is important to know when to call for help when the situation
demands.

Local anaesthesia is widely used in the ED, and is one of the
skills foundation trainees learn in the early days. It is
comparatively safe if the doctor is aware of how to perform the

procedure and the upper limit of the dose for a particular patient.

Finally, conscious sedation is also widely used in the ED for reducing fractures and/or dislocations and minor operations. However, it carries the same risks as GA and should be carried out by a doctor who is trained in the procedure as well as in resuscitation. A risk assessment should be performed as a patient with high risks (previous cardiac or respiratory diseases) must be sedated with extreme caution. In addition, sedation should be used with great care in elderly people, and in children, as the required dosage is often much lower than in adults.

This chapter mainly covers the issues surrounding analgesia, local anaesthesia, and risk assessment. ■

1. A 38-year-old man accidently stubbs his toe against a door. He is in pain. His toes are shown in Fig. 7.1.

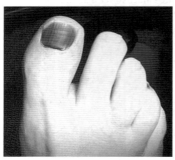

Which is the *single* most immediate, effective way of managing his pain? ★

A Codeine phosphate

B Digital nerve block

C Paracetamol

D Pressure dressings

E Trephining

2. An 85-year-old man has been having severe upper abdominal pain since this morning. He has AF, hypertension, and generalized arthritis. He takes a variety of medications. Which *single* drug is most likely to be the cause of this pain? ★

A Codeine phosphate

B Digoxin

C Nifedipine

D Piroxicam

E Warfarin

3. A 25-year-old man had a laceration on his index finger, which was repaired under a digital block using 3mL of 1% lidocaine. He asks how long it will take for the sensation to return. Which is the *single* most likely time? ★

A 20min

B 45min

C 75min

D 90min

E 120min

4. A 45-year-old man has a laceration on his right forearm, which requires suturing under 1% lidocaine. He weighs 75kg. Which is the *single* most appropriate maximum dose of lidocaine that should be used? ★

A 16mL

B 18mL

C 20mL

D 22mL

E 25mL

5. A 25-year-old man is having an injection of 1% lidocaine in his finger in preparation for the repair of a laceration. He starts feeling numbness around his mouth and tongue. Which is the *single* most appropriate action to take immediately? ★

A Monitor and carry on

B Reassure and carry on

C Stop the procedure and give diazepam

D Stop the procedure and give oxygen

E Stop the procedure and give rebreathing bag

6. A 25-year-old man has been brought to the emergency department after being involved in a road traffic collision. He is on treatment for indigestion and is allergic to opioids. The upper part of his left thigh is obviously deformed and he is in severe pain. Which is the *single* most immediate effective way of managing the pain? ★ ★

A Codeine phosphate IM

B Diclofenac rectal

C Elevate the leg

D Femoral nerve block

E Plaster of Paris back slab

7. A 25 year old man has had a fall. His X-ray is shown in Fig. 7.2. A haematoma block using 1% lidocaine has been planned for reduction.

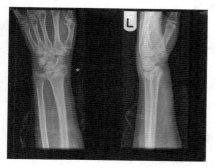

Which is the *single* contraindication to performing a haematoma block? ★ ★ ★

A Five-day old injury

B Inability to move the fingers

C Large swelling on the dorsum of the wrist

D Tingling in the thumb and index finger

E Weakness of the little finger

8. A 75-year-old man has dislocated his right shoulder, which requires reduction under sedation. He has stable angina and been smoking 25 cigarettes per day for the past 50 years. He is an active and independent person. His risk of developing perioperative complications is being assessed using the ASA classification of disease severity. Which is the *single* most appropriate score? ★ ★ ★

A 1

B 2

C 3

D 4

E 5

Analgesia and anaesthesia

ANALGESIA AND ANAESTHESIA
ANSWERS

Single Best Answers

1. B ★ OHEM, 4th edn →pp280–1

The patient has a subungual haematoma, which is very painful and caused by a build-up of pressure from the collection of blood underneath the nail in a limited space. It may be associated with a fracture of the underlying terminal phalanx. The best way of providing pain relief is to perform a digital nerve block, which involves injecting 1% lidocaine at the base of the toe on both the lateral and medial sides.

A and C: Analgesics may be prescribed but are not as effective as the digital block.

D: Pressure dressing may make the pain worse. There is already pressure under the nail bed because of accumulated blood contributing to pain.

E: Trephining (draining the haematoma by trephining the nail, which is done by applying gentle pressure with the tip of a red-hot needle or straightened paper clip) is an effective method of pain relief in such a situation if there is no underlying distal phalangeal fracture. The digital nerve block in comparison is effective in both soft tissue injuries and fractures.

2. D ★ OHEM, 4th edn →p283

NSAIDs can cause gastric irritation, diarrhoea, GI bleeding, and perforation; the risk is increased at higher drug dosages and in patients aged >60 years and those with a history of peptic ulcers. All NSAIDs can have serious adverse effects, but ibuprofen, diclofenac, and naproxen are relatively safe and cover most requirements. Ibuprofen has the lowest incidence of side effects. When possible, advise taking NSAIDs after food to reduce the risk of GI side effects. If treatment with NSAIDs is essential in patients with high risk of GI problems consider prophylactic treatment with proton pump inhibitors.

3. B ★   OHEM, 4th edn →pp290–1, 297

Lidocaine is the local anaesthetic used most often for local infiltration and for nerve blocks. It is available in 0.5%, 1%, and 2% solutions, either plain (without adrenaline (epinephrine)) or with adrenaline 1:200 000. For routine use the most suitable choice is 1% plain lidocaine. Lidocaine acts within 1–2min and the effects last for 30–60min for plain lidocaine and up to 90min for lidocaine with adrenaline. The duration of action varies with the dosage and the status of the local circulation.

There are various types of block where lidocaine may be used:

- Local infiltration: used most often in the ED; the local anaesthetic is injected subcutaneously in the immediate area of the wound.
- Field block: this involves infiltration of local anaesthetic around the operative field; it used in the ED for dirty and ragged wounds, and cleaning gravel abrasions. Sometimes a large volume of the agent is required, so check the maximum safe dose and use 0.5% solution or lidocaine with adrenaline to increase the amount of required local anaesthetic.
- Digital block: this involves anaesthetizing the digital nerves in the fingers and toes.
- Nerve blocks in the wrist or ankle block specific nerves to allow operating on the hand or foot, respectively.
- Haematoma block: this is infiltration of the local anaesthetic into the fracture haematoma before manipulation of Colles' fracture.

4. D ★   OHEM, 4th edn →p291

The dose of lidocaine to be used is 3mg/kg body weight, which in this case is 225mg, i.e. 22.5mL. So the nearest maximum safest dose is 22mL. Ideally the dose required is the minimum that would anaesthetize the area, so the full maximum dose is often not required.

5. D ★   OHEM, 4th edn →p292

Toxic effects result from overdose of local anaesthetics or inadvertent IV injections, and the first symptoms and signs are usually neurological, with numbness of the mouth and tongue, slurring of speech, light-headedness, tinnitus, confusion, and drowsiness. Muscle twitching, convulsions, and coma can also occur. Cardiovascular toxicity may initially result in tachycardia and hypertension, and later there is hypotension with bradycardia and heart block. Ventricular arrhythmias and cardiac arrest occur occasionally, especially with bupivacaine. Toxic effects may start immediately if an IV injection is given.

The treatment of toxicity is to stop the procedure immediately, get *senior* help, clear and maintain the airway, give 100% oxygen, obtain IV access, move the patient to the resuscitation room, monitor the ECG, and record the pulse, BP, respiratory rate, and conscious level. Treatment with lipid emulsion may be considered with senior guidance.

6. D ★★   OHEM, 4th edn →pp312–3

A femoral nerve block, which is obtained by giving local anaesthetic injection in the femoral triangle, is an effective way of achieving pain control and should be done even before the patient goes for X-rays. In adults, the block is usually given by using a mixture of 5mL of 1% lidocaine and 5mL of 0.5% bupivacaine. Insert a 21G needle, with a syringe attached and containing the above mixture, perpendicular to the skin and 1cm lateral to the femoral artery pulsation in the femoral triangle to a depth of about 3cm. If paraesthesiae occur, withdraw the needle by 2–3mm. Aspirate and check the syringe for blood. Inject the local anaesthetic mixture while moving the needle up and down, fanning out laterally to about 3cm from the artery. This procedure is performed by a senior person experienced in doing femoral nerve blocks (OHEM, 4th edn pp302–3). This is safer and more effective if done under US guidance by an appropriately-trained person.

A: Codeine phosphate is contraindicated as it an opioid.

B: The patient possibly has a displaced fracture of his femoral shaft. As he has a history of indigestion, diclofenac should not be used. Moreover, a suppository would be awkward to apply because of the pain and fracture.

C: Simple elevation is not helpful, as any movement will increase the pain. However, using a traction splint (e.g. Thomas' splint) with mild elevation may help in reducing the pain by immobilizing the limb.

E. A back slab is not helpful, it is also cumbersome to apply and will cause more pain.

7. A ★★★   OHEM, 4th edn →p297

A Colles' fracture can be manipulated after infiltration of local anaesthetic in the fracture haematoma and around the ulnar styloid. Contraindications and precautions include: fractures >24h old, since the organization of haematoma would prevent spread of the local anaesthetic agent; infection of the skin over the fracture; methaemoglobinaemia (avoid prilocaine, as when it is used in excess of 400mg, one of its metabolites, hydroxylated *O*-toluidine, reduces oxyhaemoglobin and resulting in formation of methaemoglobin, and thus may cause methaemoglobinaemia).

Wildsmith JAW, Armitage EN (eds) (1993) *Principles and Practice of Regional Anaesthesia*, 2nd edn. London: Churchill Livingstone, p63.

8. B ★★★ OHEM, 4th edn →pp318–9

The ASA classification is widely used in EDs to ascertain the risks of potential complications of conscious sedation or short GA for small procedures. It depends on the patient's comorbidity status.

1. Healthy patient with no systemic disease. (General perioperative mortality of 0.05%.)
2. Patient with mild to moderate disease, which does not limit their activity in any way. (General perioperative mortality of 0.4%.)
3. Patient with severe systemic disturbances from any cause, which limits activity (ischaemic heart disease, severe chronic pulmonary obstructive disease, etc.). (General perioperative mortality of 4.5%.)
4. Patient with a severe systemic disease with constant threat to life (severe COPD, advanced liver disease, etc.). (General perioperative mortality of 25%.)
5. Moribund patient who is unlikely to survive 24h with or without surgery. (General perioperative mortality of 50%.)

Extremes of age, smoking, and pregnancy are criteria for ASA 2.

Cooper N, Forrest K, Cramp P (2006) *Essential Guide to Acute Care*, 2nd edn. Oxford: Blackwell, p152.

Analgesia and anaesthesia

CHAPTER 8

MAJOR TRAUMA

'The creative person is usually rebellious. He or she is the survivor of a trauma called education.'

Anon

In the UK, trauma is currently the commonest cause of death in people <40 years and its incidence is predicted to rise over the next 20 years. So you have an important role in the assessment and management of this group of patients.

Doctors of the ED perform a vital role in the early stages of management of trauma patients. In patients with multiple injuries, the care is delivered by a trauma team constituted by middle-grade doctors from various specialties. A senior doctor, usually from the ED and with training in dealing with trauma, leads the team. The trauma team is often requested by the prehospital ambulance personnel, but this is not always the case. Although in your first few days you would not be expected to manage such situations on your own, you may come across a patient with serious trauma behind the curtains in a cubicle. Recognizing the seriousness of the situation and calling for help in the form of a trauma team may make all the difference to that patient in terms of recovery.

The principles of assessment and management of trauma patients are discussed in the first answer of this chapter. The ATLS course introduces you to the principles of early management of trauma victims and this can be applied to any trauma patient whom you will see in the ED. The skills you learn on the ATLS course are applicable in many situations. It is advisable to attend this training course while you are working in the ED.

You should suspect major trauma in the following situations:

- Related to vehicles: high-speed collisions, victim's ejection from the vehicle (partial or total), rollover, prolonged extrication, etc.
- Death of a co-passenger

- Pedestrians run over or thrown away to a distance, or with a significant impact (>20mph/32kph)
- Falls from a height of >6m in adults and >3m in children or two to three times the height of the child.

Resuscitation in the first hour in the resuscitation room has been proved to reduce mortality and morbidity among trauma patients, and so it might be you who will have saved the life of an individual. ■

SINGLE BEST ANSWERS

1. A 20-year-old woman lost control of her car and hit a tree while driving at the speed of 60mph. She has a large laceration on the parietal scalp, and some bruises on the right chest wall. Her GCS score is 14/15 and she is speaking in sentences. She has been given high-flow oxygen via a facemask. Which is the *single* most appropriate immediate management? ★

A Cervical spine immobilization

B Chest tube insertion

C CT scan of brain

D Endotracheal intubation

E IV access

2. A 35-year-old man skidded on a wet road while riding his motorbike at a speed of 70mph (112kmph). He has a large haematoma on the temporal scalp, some bruises on the right chest wall and abdomen, and a deformed right thigh. His GCS score is 11/15. He has been given high-flow oxygen via a facemask. Which is the *single* most immediate radiological investigation required during the initial resuscitation phase? ★

A CT of the abdomen

B CT of the brain

C X-ray of the abdomen

D X-ray of the chest

E X-ray of the femur

3. A 29-year-old man was driving at 60mph (96kmph) without a seat belt when his car was involved in a head-on collision with an oncoming car. He has been immobilized on a spinal board. The pain around his chest becomes worse when he tries to talk. He has bruising on the right side of the chest. His heart rate is 110bpm, BP 100/80mmHg, and respiratory rate 32breaths/min. He is on 15L of oxygen via a mask and receiving warm normal saline through two grey cannulae. His chest X-ray is shown in Fig. 8.1.

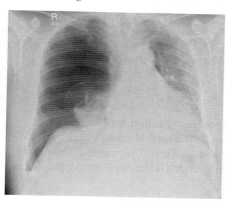

Which is the *single* most appropriate immediate step? ★

A Chest tube insertion

B CT scan of chest

C Endotracheal intubation

D Needle decompression

E Paracetamol IV

4. A 22-year-old man fell from his motorbike after skidding on an icy road. He responds to pain and responds incoherently when asked questions. His heart rate is 46bpm, BP 152/94mmHg, respiratory rate 12breathes/min, and oxygen saturation 94%. The diameter of the left pupil is 5mm and of the right is 2mm. He is receiving oxygen and IV normal saline. Which is the *single* most likely underlying mechanism for his condition? ★

A Excessive IV fluid administration

B Hypercarbia (hypercapnia) following poor ventilation

C Hypovolaemia with cerebral hypoperfusion

D Hypoxia following reduced oxygenation

E Increased ICP

5. A 28-year-old man has been bitten by his dog. He has continuous brisk bleeding from his right distal forearm and wrist area. His pulse is 120bpm and BP 100/78mmHg. Which is the *single* most appropriate immediate step? ★

A Apply direct pressure to the wound

B Attach to cardiac monitor

C Call the surgeons immediately

D Give O-negative blood

E Give 1L of normal saline stat

6. A 20-year-old man was involved in a pub fight after drinking 7 pints of lager. On arrival at the ED, he opens his eyes to verbal command, makes occasional disorientated comments when asked questions, and squeezes his fingers when asked to do so. His heart rate is 70bpm, BP 110/60mmHg, and respiratory rate 20breaths/min. Which is the *single* most appropriate management? ★

A Arranging for definitive airway followed by imaging

B Arranging imaging after immobilizing the cervical spine

C Discharging him with a relative to sleep off the alcohol at home

D Leaving him as he will wake up later when the alcohol wears off

E Monitoring in the left lateral decubitus position until he wakes up

7. A 20-year-old man accidentally burnt himself when sitting very near a camp fire. He has blistering and peeling of the skin of the scrotum and a 2cm patch on his penis. His heart rate is 100/min, BP 110/80mmHg, and respiratory rate 22breaths/min. The wound has been dressed and he is being given high-flow oxygen. After appropriate analgesia, which is the *single* most appropriate management? ★

A Follow-up in the ED

B Follow-up by the patient's GP

C Referral to burn centre

D Referral to burns outpatients

E Referral to general surgeons

8. A 20-year-old man was sleeping when his house caught fire. He woke up coughing, and on his way out his clothes caught fire. He has blistering and peeling of the skin of his face, with some black soot around his central facial area. He is alert but finding it difficult to talk. He has a cough with blackish sputum. His heart rate is 100bpm, BP 110/80mmHg, and respiratory rate 24breaths/min. He has been given high-flow oxygen and his SaO_2 is 100% on air. Which is the *single* most appropriate initial management? ★

A Applying dressing on the face

B Arranging a chest X-ray

C Establishing a definitive airway

D Giving IM analgesia

E Transfer to burns centre

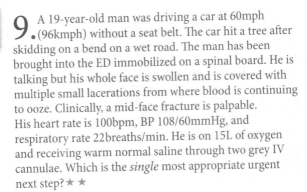

9. A 19-year-old man was driving a car at 60mph (96kmph) without a seat belt. The car hit a tree after skidding on a bend on a wet road. The man has been brought into the ED immobilized on a spinal board. He is talking but his whole face is swollen and is covered with multiple small lacerations from where blood is continuing to ooze. Clinically, a mid-face fracture is palpable. His heart rate is 100bpm, BP 108/60mmHg, and respiratory rate 22breaths/min. He is on 15L of oxygen and receiving warm normal saline through two grey IV cannulae. Which is the *single* most appropriate urgent next step? ★ ★

A CT scan of the face

B Endotracheal intubation

C Prophylactic surgical airway

D Suturing of the facial lacerations

E Trauma series X-rays

10. An 18-year-old woman has stabbed herself at the right side of the lower part of her neck in an suicidal attempt. There is a 3cm long, deep wound just above the sternoclavicular joint. Her heart rate is 100bpm, BP 110/70mmHg, respiratory rate 22breaths/min, and oxygen saturation 100% on 15L of oxygen. She is alert and has pain at the site of the injury. Which is the *single* most appropriate treatment position? ★ ★

A 20° prop-up position

B 45° prop-up position

C Head down position

D No special position

E Supine position

11. A 41-year-old woman has sustained self-inflicted burns to her whole body by igniting herself after pouring white spirit. Her legs are shown in Fig. 8.2.

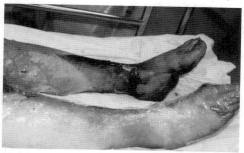

Which is the *single* most appropriate, urgent treatment for the left lower leg burns? ★ ★

A Amputation

B Bandage dressing

C Debridement of the wound

D Escharotomy

E Skin grafting

12. A 22-year-old man has been brought to the ED following a road traffic collision. He has multiple lacerations on various parts of the body, bilateral pulmonary contusions, and rupture of the surface of the spleen. What is his *single* most appropriate ISS? ★ ★ ★ ★

A 18

B 26

C 28

D 32

E 35

13. A 28-year-old man has bruising and pain in his upper abdomen following a road traffic collision. His pulse rate is 120bpm, BP 88/45mmHg, and respiratory rate 28breaths/min. He is on 15L of oxygen and there is IV normal saline running through two large-bore cannulae. Which is the *single* most appropriate immediate investigation? ★ ★ ★

A Abdominal X-ray

B CT scan of abdomen

C DPL

D Focused ultrasound scan

E Urgent laparoscopy

14. A 28-year-old man has bruising and pain in the abdomen following a road traffic collision. His pulse rate is 120bpm, BP 86/48mmHg, and respiratory rate 30breaths/min. He is on 15L of oxygen and has IV crystalloids running through two large-bore cannulae. A FAST scan taken in the ED is positive for intra-abdominal fluid. What is the *single* most likely minimum amount of fluid present in the abdomen? ★ ★ ★ ★

A 100mL

B 200mL

C 300mL

D 400mL

E 500mL

15. A 68-year-old man has bruising and pain in the chest from the seat belt following a road traffic collision. He has no other injury. His pulse rate is 70bpm, BP 148/90mmHg, and respiratory rate 20breaths/min. The ECG and chest X-ray are normal. His sternal X-ray is shown in Fig. 8.3.

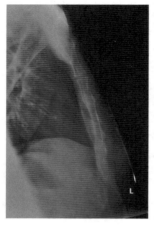

What is the *single* most appropriate management? ★ ★ ★ ★

A Admitting to coronary care unit for observation

B Arranging outpatient 24-h ECG recording

C CT scan of the chest

D Discharge with analgesics

E Open reduction with internal fixation

16. A 30-year-old man was sleeping when his house caught fire. He woke up coughing severely and short of breath. While trying to escape his clothes caught fire. He collapsed and died on his way to hospital. His face was covered with black soot. Which is the *single* most likely causative agent/s for his death? ★ ★ ★

A Ammonia

B CO

C Hydrogen cyanide

D Ketones/aldehydes

E Sulphur oxides

17. A 21-year-old man has been brought to the ED in the early hours of the morning. He was found lying on a footpath for an unknown period of time near the front entrance of a nightclub. He might have been involved in a fight with a gang, receiving multiple injuries. He had been drinking alcohol in the past few hours and possibly has taken recreational drugs. On arrival he opens his eyes on verbal command. He is covered with many bruises around his shoulders, back, arms, and lower limbs. He has severe pain in his back and limbs. His temperature is 37°C, heart rate 100bpm, BP 140/85mmHg, respiratory rate 24breaths/min and SaO$_2$ 97% on air. X-rays of his chest, scapulae, humerus, and spine are normal. Which is the *single* most important life-threatening diagnosis to consider? ★ ★ ★

A Alcohol intoxication

B Chest injuries

C Compartment syndrome

D Crush syndrome

E Ecstasy poisoning

18. A 41-year-old woman has back and neck pain following a road traffic collision. She has been immobilized by the ambulance crew on a spinal board. Her heart rate is 120bpm, BP 91/70mmHg, respiratory rate 28breaths/min, and GCS score 12/15. Which is the *single most* appropriate next step? ★ ★ ★

A Leave her on the board and send for X-rays

B Leave her on the board until the primary survey is done

C Remove the board by lifting the patient up with the help of nurses and doctors

D Remove the board by log roll method before the primary survey

E Remove the straps and ask the patient to roll to one side so that the board can be removed

19. A 78-year-old man had a fall and hit his head on the banister. He also lost consciousness for a few minutes. He has had one episode of vomiting. He has been taking warfarin for the past few years for AF. He is now opening his eyes to pain, obeying commands, and making confused conversation. He has a large bruise on the left side of the head. His INR is 4.5. Which is the *single* most appropriate initial management? ★ ★ ★ ★

A Admitting for neuro-observation under the orthopaedics team

B Arranging brain CT scan

C Arranging skull X-ray

D Discharging him with head injury advice

E Referring to the neurosurgeons

20. A 22-year-old man has accidentally caught fire in his kitchen. He has redness on the front of the neck and chest. He has blistering and peeling of the skin on the front of both upper limbs. Which is the *single* most likely total area involved? ★ ★ ★ ★

A 9%

B 13.5%

C 15%

D 18%

E 22.5%

MAJOR TRAUMA
ANSWERS

Single Best Answers

1. **A** ★   OHEM, 4th edn → pp328–29

Cervical spine control is the first priority in a patient who may have spine injury. Anybody with a reduced GCS score and the possibility of distraction injury must have their cervical spine protected while assessing and protecting the airway at the beginning of the primary survey.

This patient's GCS is 14/15 and she is talking; therefore, she does not require immediate intubation/anaesthetist's help at this stage. She should be managed by the trauma team, which should include various specialists, i.e. ED physician, anaesthetist, surgeon, orthopaedic surgeon, and radiologist. She will require IV access as a part of assessment and management of the circulation, which comes after managing problems of airway (with cervical spine control) and breathing. She will also require a chest X-ray and if required, insertion of chest tube.

According to ATLS, treatment of all patients with major trauma involves the same phases:

- Primary survey
- Resuscitation phase
- Secondary survey
- Definitive care phase.

On initial reception of a seriously injured patient, life-threatening problems are identified and addressed as rapidly as possible. An ABCDE approach is adopted, with each of the following aspects being quickly evaluated and treated:

- A – Airway maintenance and cervical spine control
- B – Breathing and ventilation
- C – Circulation and haemorrhage control
- D – Disability (rapid assessment of neurological status)
- E – Exposure (the patient is completely undressed to allow full examination).

American College of Surgeons Committee on Trauma (2008)
Advanced Trauma Life Support for Doctors, Student Course Manual,
8th edn. American College of Surgeons, pp2–5.

2. D ★   OHEM, 4th edn → p330

To detect any major life-threatening injuries X-rays of the chest and
pelvis are obligatory during the initial resuscitation, while carrying
out primary survey. A cross-table lateral cervical spine film may also
be requested at this stage.

X-ray of femur may be done once the patient is stabilized. There is
no place for abdomen or skull X-rays during primary survey. As the
patient has external evidence of abdominal injury, he may need a
CT scan later, once the primary survey is done and the life-
threatening conditions have been dealt with. A shocked or unstable
patient must not be taken to a CT scanner as it is often called the
'doughnut of death'.

American College of Surgeons Committee on Trauma (2008)
Advanced Trauma Life Support for Doctors, Student Course Manual,
8th edn. American College of Surgeons, p118.

3. D ★   OHEM, 4th edn → p338

The patient has a right-sided tension pneumothorax pushing the
mediastinum to the opposite side. His BP is low with a tachycardia.
Movement of the mediastinum leads to kinking of the great vessels,
thereby reducing venous return and cardiac output. Additional
compromise results from compression of the lung on the opposite
side. The process leading to tension pneumothorax may occur very
rapidly, culminating in cardiac arrest within minutes. This is most
often a clinical diagnosis and such patients should not wait for an
X-ray of the chest for the above reason. Therefore, the immediate
step would be insertion of a wide-bore IV cannula in the right
second intercostal space, in the mid-clavicular line, to release the
pressure. Needle decompression averts the emergency for about
20–30min, during which time a chest tube must be inserted.

The patient would die if he was taken to a CT scanner. The
endotracheal intubation may make the situation worse as with each
breath of positive pressure ventilation, the pneumothorax will grow
bigger, leading to cardiac arrest. Paracetamol IV can be deferred
until the emergency is dealt with.

4. E ★   OHEM, 4th edn → p370

Increased ICP produces a diminishing conscious level and causes
herniation of the temporal lobe through the tentorial hiatus,
which stretches the oculomotor nerve, resulting in ipsilateral

papillary dilatation. ICP leads to a reflex increase in systemic arterial BP together with bradycardia (Cushing's response). Options A–D would not cause these features.

Williams NS, Bulstrode CJK, O'Connell PR (eds) (2008) *Bailey and Love's Short Practice of Surgery*, 25th edn. London: Hodder Arnold, pp299–301.

5. A ★   OHEM, 4th edn → pp328–29

This patient is bleeding briskly and will be in shock if the bleeding is not stopped immediately. The simplest and most effective way to stop the bleeding is the application of direct manual pressure on the bleeding site or proximal to it, and elevation of the limb. This can be done during transit or even before reaching the resuscitation room. O-negative blood is only indicated in life-threatening severe shock. The other options are important parts of the emergency management but can be done as the next steps.

6. B ★   OHEM, 4th edn → p370

The patient's GCS score is 13/15 (E3, V4, M6). He does not require definitive airway. Note down if the patient smells of alcohol, but *never* assume that a reduced GCS score is because of alcohol. Such patients may go for imaging and/or be admitted for neuro-observation. Because of the possibility of cervical spine injury, the patient must not be left in the left lateral decubitus position until such injury has been excluded. Prior to examination to rule out the neck injury, the patient must not be under the influence of alcohol and must be fully conscious.

7. C ★   OHEM, 4th edn → p406

Burns in the genitalia area should be referred to a burn specialist. Indications for referring patients to a burn specialist are:

- Airway burns
- Significant full thickness burns, especially over joints
- Burns >10%
- Burns in special areas (hands, face, perineum, feet).

8. C   OHEM, 4th edn → pp333–5

Signs of upper airway problems (facial burns, stridor, dysphagia, drooling, or reduced consciousness) indicate an urgent need for early tracheal intubation by an experienced doctor (ED, ICU, or anaesthesia) with appropriate training. Large burns on the face are difficult to cover with dressings and so may be left open and cleaned regularly. IM analgesia is unpredictable and ineffective in extensive burns. Chest X-ray may be done after protection of the airway.

Such patients should be transferred to a burns centre after securing the airway.

Tetanus vaccine (a booster dose or initiation of a course) may be given but is not urgent.

→ www.toxbase.org/Poisons-Index-A-Z/S-Products/Smoke-Inhalation/

9. B ★★ OHEM, 4th edn → pp380–3

A severely injured person would die very soon unless efforts are made to ensure oxygenated blood reaches the brain and other vital organs. Clear, maintain, and protect the airway, ensure the ventilation is adequate, and give oxygen in as high a concentration as possible.

Facial trauma demands aggressive airway management. Trauma to the midface can result in fractures and dislocations that compromise the nasopharynx and the oropharynx. Such patients require intubation and ventilation urgently, before their airway becomes obstructed by soft tissue swelling.

This patient will require a CT scan of face, but after securing the airway. A surgical airway may be required if the endotracheal intubation fails. In keeping with the principles outlined by the ATLS group, trauma series X-rays should be done after management of the airway. The continuous oozing of blood is the result of multiple fractures of the facial bones, therefore, suturing the multiple small lacerations would only exacerbate the swelling. This can be dealt with following protection of the airway.

American College of Surgeons Committee on Trauma (2008) *Advanced Trauma Life Support for Doctors, Student Course Manual*, 8th edn. American College of Surgeons, p26.

10. C ★★ OHEM, 4th edn → p388

Deep stab wounds should be treated with extreme seriousness. The stab wounds in a situation such as the present scenario may be associated with injury to the internal jugular vein, which might be bleeding slowly inside. Thus, such patients should be treated in a head down position to avoid air embolism to the brain.

The neck is divided into 'zones' when classifying wounds:

- Zone 1 extends from the clavicles to the cricoid cartilage
- Zone 2 extends from the cricoid to the angle of the mandible
- Zone 3 is the area from the angle of the mandible to the skull base.

11. D ★ ★   OHEM, 4th edn → p400

On the distal third of the left leg (Fig. 8.2), the black and leathery area is a full thickness burn and it is covering the whole circumference of the leg. Such burns cause constriction of the blood vessels supplying the foot. To save the foot from vascular compromise, an escharotomy is required urgently. Escharotomy is a surgical incision into necrotic tissue resulting from a severe burn. The procedure is sometimes necessary to prevent the oedema from generating sufficient interstitial pressure that impairs capillary filling and causes ischaemia. The proximal part of the left leg has partial thickness burns (Fig. 8.2). The right leg has normal skin and partial thickness burns which have already been treated by covering with cling film.

Amputation is not an option in this scenario; every endeavour should be made to save the left leg. A bandage dressing would make the situation worse. Cling film may be used but would not solve the leg-threatening emergency. Skin grafting would be required later in a proper theatre environment. Escharotomy may be performed in the resuscitation room of the ED.

Williams NS, Bulstrode CJK, O'Connell PR (eds) (2008) *Bailey and Love's Short Practice of Surgery*, 25th edn. London: Hodder Arnold, p385.

12. B ★ ★ ★ ★   OHEM, 4th edn → p331

The ISS is widely used to score the anatomical injuries of an individual patient retrospectively. The score is obtained by first scoring each individual injury using the AIS, which attributes a score of between 1 and 6 to each individual injury, as follows:

- AIS 1 = minor injury
- AIS 2 = moderate injury
- AIS 3 = serious injury
- AIS 4 = severe injury
- AIS 5 = critical injury
- AIS 6 = inevitable fatal injury.

To calculate the ISS from an array of AIS scores for a patient, the three highest AIS scores in different body regions are squared and then added together. ISS considers the body as comprising six regions: head/neck; face; chest; abdomen; extremities; external (skin). Possible ISS scores range from 1 to 75. Any patient with an AIS of 6 is automatically given an ISS of 75.

The ISS in this patient is: $(4)^2$ (bilateral pulmonary contusions) + $(3)^2$ (spleen rupture) + $(1)^2$ (widespread multiple lacerations) = 26

→ www.trauma.org/archive/scores/iss.html

13. D ★★★ OHEM, 4th edn → p331

This patient is in shock and it will be unsafe to take the patient to the radiology department for a CT scan. DPL is an invasive test and used rarely in the UK. A focused ultrasound scan (FAST or focus assessment with sonography for trauma), done at the bedside in the ED, is the most appropriate investigation in these circumstances, and if it shows free fluid, this indicates visceral injury which may require urgent laparotomy. The abdominal X-ray has no role in such a situation.

14. E ★★★★ OHEM, 4th edn → p331

FAST scan is increasingly used in the ED resuscitation room to assess the chest and abdomen of acutely injured patients, especially those with shock. It can be performed by a trained ED doctor, surgeon, or radiologist. A positive FAST scan is one which identifies any free fluid in the abdomen or in the pericardium. Visible free fluid in the abdomen implies a minimum volume of about 500mL.

15. D ★★★★ OHEM, 4th edn → p341

Sternal fracture frequently occurs during road traffic collisions, either due to seat belt or impact against the steering wheel. The injury may be associated with myocardial contusion, or chest or spinal injuries. Patients often have anterior chest pain with localized tenderness. An ECG must be done to exclude arrhythmias, myocardial infarction, or contusion and troponins checked if there are any ECG changes. Patients may be discharged if there is an isolated sternal fracture with a normal ECG, no associated injury, and no previous cardiopulmonary dysfunction. Patients with suspected myocardial contusion or infarction may require admission to CCU. There is no place for outpatient ECG recording in this scenario. CT scan of the chest is needed if there is suspicion of chest injury on chest and/or spinal X-ray. Such fractures heal spontaneously and do not require internal fixation.

16. B ★★★ OHEM, 4th edn → p404

CO is responsible for 85% of fire deaths, though all other products of combustion mentioned above contribute to bronchospasm and mucosal injury.

Ammonia is a strong alkali which is highly soluble in water and causes chemical burns. Exposure by any route (inhalation, ingestion, skin exposure, splashes in the eyes) may be dangerous.
Hydrogen cyanide (prussic acid) is a gas with many commercial uses, particularly in synthetic fibre manufacture and fumigation.

Poisoning with hydrogen cyanide most often occurs in petroleum refinery and sewage storage tank workers. It is extremely toxic after inhalation and ingestion. Tissue hypoxia occurs within minutes, causing dysfunction of central nervous system and heart.

Ketones/aldehydes may be formed following oxidation of alcohol (e.g. methanol) in the body in acute poisoning causing toxicity. Sulphur oxide is a non-flammable, colourless gas with a pungent odour, and is used as a preservative, disinfectant and bleach. It is irritating to the eyes and the respiratory system.

→ www.toxbase.org

17. D ★ ★ ★   OHEM, 4th edn → p408

The patient has crush syndrome. Alcohol intoxication will cause an altered sensorium. The compartment syndrome in the arms (very rare) will cause pain, mainly locally. Ecstasy poisoning may cause a high temperature but is also a precipitating factor for the crush syndrome. Fractures of multiple bones have already been excluded by X-rays. Always have a high level of suspicion in such circumstances and arrange appropriate investigations.

In crush syndrome, prolonged crushing of the muscles releases myoglobin and vasoactive substances into the circulation. It also reduces the blood volume by sequestration of many litres of fluid, resulting in renal vasoconstriction and ischaemia. The released myoglobin may cause renal tubular obstruction. The condition should be treated with aggressive fluid resuscitation (saline 1–1.5L/h in adults) as soon as it is recognized. Urine output should be closely monitored after catheterization.

Williams NS, Bulstrode CJK, O'Connell PR (eds) (2008) *Bailey and Love's Short Practice of Surgery*, 25th edn. London: Hodder Arnold, p423.

18. B ★ ★ ★   OHEM, 4th edn → pp390–1

Usually patients with multiple injuries or suspicion of spinal injury will have been transported on a spinal board, which should be removed as soon as the primary survey is completed and resuscitation commenced. Remove the board before X-rays if possible as it may affect the quality of the images. As the patient is in shock, she needs immediate primary survey and resuscitation; the log-roll can be done after the patient is reasonably stable. It is unsafe to ask the patient to roll as she is in shock and there is suspicion of spinal injuries.

19. B ★ ★ ★ ★ OHEM, 4th edn → p372

According to NICE guidelines, the patient has a depressed GCS, and as he is on warfarin, he needs an urgent CT brain scan. Skull X-rays are unhelpful in such circumstances. Patient must not be discharged without appropriate investigation, and without making a definitive diagnosis following a brain scan. It is not appropriate to refer to a neurosurgeon.

→ www.nice.org.uk/nicemedia/pdf/CG56QuickRedGuide.pdf

20. A ★ ★ ★ ★ OHEM, 4th edn → pp400–1

Fig. 8.4 shows the Lund and Browder charts that are used for assessing the extent of burns.

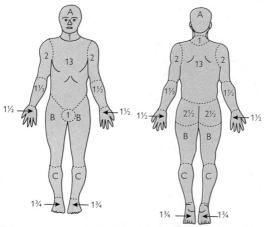

Relative percentage of area affected by growth (age in years)

	0	1	5	10	15	Adult
A: half of head	9½	8½	6½	5½	4½	3½
B: half of thigh	2¾	3½	4	4½	4½	4¾
C: half of leg	2½	9½	2¾	3	3¼	3½

Adult rule of nines (ignore the erythema only):

- Head = 9%
- Each arm = 9%
- Each leg = 18%
- Front of trunk = 18%

- Back of trunk = 18%
- Perineum = 1%

According to the adult rule of nines, the front of both the upper limbs will be 4.5×2 = 9%. To estimate rapidly, the palmer surface of the patient's palm (not including the fingers) represents approximately 0.75% body surface area. The erythema in the front of the neck and chest does not count towards the calculation.

For more information, see *Emergencies in Primary Care*, pp230–1.

CHAPTER 9

WOUNDS, FRACTURES, ORTHOPAEDICS

'To him whose feet hurt, everything hurts'

Socrates

A significant number of patients attending the ED are those who are often referred to as 'minors', 'streamers', 'walking wounded', etc. These include patients with minor injuries, wounds, fractures or other soft tissue injuries. Therefore, a basic knowledge of anatomy and its application in various circumstances is mandatory. The injuries mentioned above are rarely life-threatening, but they may be limb-threatening and severely disabling. So it is extremely important to avoid errors in diagnosis and management, and to know when to ask for help at the appropriate time.

By following the key principles listed below, you will be able to avoid many problems with such patients:

- In the history, a detailed description of the mechanism of injury and the patient's complaint will help in predicting the type of injury sustained.

- A careful and thorough physical examination can point to the site and type of injury, on the basis of which appropriate radiological images can then be requested.

- A neurovascular examination must be completed and documented in every limb injury, before and after any reductions, and before and after immobilization.

- Appropriate radiological imaging, accompanied by a thorough physical examination, can pick up injuries with a high degree of accuracy. Inadequate radiographic films should not be accepted.

- Immobilize the patient if a fracture is clinically suspected even if the X-rays are negative.

- In cases of dislocations or subluxations, X-rays should be done before and after reductions, except when a delay could be potentially harmful to the patient (for example, when a severe traumatic deformity of a joint threatens to jeopardize the viability of the overlying skin).

- The patient should be able to mobilize safely before being discharged from the ED.

- Patients should be given proper aftercare instructions before leaving the ED, including how to look after themselves and to recognize limb-threatening features, the follow-up arrangement, and to return if things go wrong.

- Ask for senior help if you are not sure about an injury or its management.

Adapted from Geiderman JM, Katz D (2010) General principles of orthopaedic injuries. In: Marx JA, *et al.* (eds) *Rosen's Emergency Medicine: Concepts and Clinical Practice*, 7th edn. Philadelphia: Mosby/Elsevier, p467. ∎

SINGLE BEST ANSWERS

1. A 20-year-old woman has attended the ED after treading on a glass piece. She has a laceration of about 2cm on the left big toe, which is oozing blood. Which is the *single* most appropriate method to close the wound? ★

A Delayed closure

B Glue

C Neighbour strapping

D Steri-Strips

E Suturing

2. A 18-year-old man has a laceration about 5cm long on the sole of his left foot after treading on a piece of glass 12h earlier at a construction site. An X-ray of the foot does not show any glass in the wound. Which is the *single* most appropriate time of wound closure? ★

A Delay by 2–3 days

B Delay by 3–5 days

C Delay by 7 days

D Delay by 2 weeks

E Immediate closure

3. A 78-year-old woman has attended the ED after banging her right leg against a piece of furniture a few hours ago. Fig. 9.1 shows the injury on her right shin.

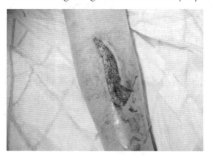

Which is the *single* most appropriate immediate treatment? ★

A Glue

B Skin grafting

C Staples

D Steri-Strips

E Suturing

4. A 47-year-old man cut his right hand while laying a carpet yesterday evening. He says that he had a tetanus booster 5 years ago and full childhood immunization. Which is the *single* most appropriate management? ★

A Giving a booster dose of anti-tetanus vaccine only

B Giving a dose of anti-tetanus immunoglobulin only

C Giving a dose of anti-tetanus vaccine and anti-tetanus immunoglobulin

D Giving a dose of anti-tetanus vaccine followed by further doses by the GP

E No action required with regards to tetanus prophylaxis

5. A 35-year-old man cut his right hand while gardening yesterday evening but he continued to finish his planting. He is fully immunized against tetanus. Which is the *single* most appropriate management option with regard to tetanus prophylaxis? ★

A A booster dose of anti-tetanus vaccine followed by completion of the course

B A booster dose of anti-tetanus vaccine only

C A booster dose of vaccine followed by anti-tetanus immunoglobulin

D A dose of anti-tetanus immunoglobulin

E No action required with regards to tetanus prophylaxis

6. A 15-year-old girl has been bitten by her dog on the left cheek. She has a laceration of about 1.5×0.5cm Which is the *single* most appropriate management? ★

A Irrigating the wound and covering with a plaster

B Irrigating the wound followed by primary closure with glue

C Irrigating the wound followed by primary closure with sutures

D Leaving the wound open and giving antibiotics

E Leaving the wound open and reviewing next day

7. A 20-year-old woman has attended the ED after accidentally cutting her right thumb while chopping vegetables. She has a laceration of about 3cm, which is bleeding briskly. Which is the *single* most appropriate management? ★

A Applying glue to seal the wound edges

B Applying tourniquet and leaving it for 45min

C Clipping the bleeding points blindly with artery forceps

D Elevating the limb after applying local pressure

E Performing digital block using lidocaine with epinephrine

8. A 40-year-old man fell on his outstretched right hand. His right elbow is very painful and deformed. Which is the *single* most important next step? ★

A Examining the elbow movements

B Examining the radial nerve

C Examining the radial pulse

D Examining the shoulder

E Palpating the fingers for tenderness

9. A 35-year-old man injured his left shoulder while making a tackle during a rugby game. His X-ray is shown in Fig. 9.2.

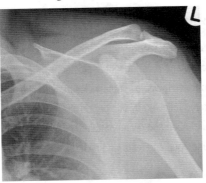

Which *single* nerve is most likely to be injured? ★

A Axillary

B Lateral pectoral

C Median

D Subscapular

E Ulnar

10. An 80-year-old man has had a fall. His left lower limb is shortened and internally rotated with flexion and adduction at the hip joint. He had a left total hip replacement 2 weeks ago. Which is the *single* most appropriate clinical sign of significant nerve damage? ★

A Inability to dorsiflex the foot

B Inability to extend the knee

C Inability to flex the hip

D Loss of sensation in the femoral triangle

E Loss of sensation over the lateral surface of the thigh

11. An 84-year-old woman has had a fall. She is distressed and has 'gone off her feet'. She is reluctant to move the right lower limb. Which is the *single* most urgent management? ★

A Applying traction

B Giving analgesia

C Referring to orthopaedics

D Referring to social services

E Send for X-ray

12. A 20-year-old man had a twisting injury of his knee while playing football a few hours earlier. The knee is now swollen and he is unable to weightbear. A medial collateral ligament injury is suspected. Which *single* clinical test is most likely to be positive? ★

A Anterior draw test

B Patellar tap

C Straight leg raise

D Valgus stress

E Varus stress

13. A 25-year-old man injured the lateral side of his left knee after receiving a kick while playing football. He has swelling, bruising, and tenderness near the upper end of the fibula. Damage to the common peroneal nerve is suspected. Which *single* clinical sign is most likely to be present if the nerve is damaged? ★

A Inability to plantarflex the foot

B Inability to plantarflex the toes

C Reduced ankle jerk

D Reduced sensation on the lateral side of the foot

E Reduced sensation on the sole

14. A 40-year-old woman slips on ice and twists her ankle (Fig. 9.3). Which is the *single* most appropriate immediate clinical examination that must be done? ★

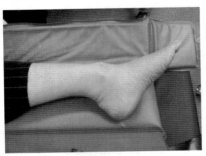

A Checking the colour of the foot

B Checking the movements of the ankle

C Checking the movements of the toes

D Checking the pulsation in the foot

E Checking the sensation of the foot

15. A 35-year-old man slipped on a kerb while walking and twisted his ankle with inward rotation of the foot. He has mild swelling, bruising, and tenderness distal to the lateral malleolus. He is able to weightbear. Which is the *single* most likely ligament injured? ★

A Anterior talofibular ligament

B Calcaneofibular ligament

C Deltoid ligament

D Inferior tibiofibular ligament

E Transverse ligament

16. A 60-year-old woman slipped yesterday while going downstairs. She twisted her ankle, rotating the foot inwards. She has tenderness, swelling, and bruising on the lateral aspect of the foot. The foot X-ray is shown in Fig. 9.4. Which is the *single* most likely tendon involved in the mechanism? ★

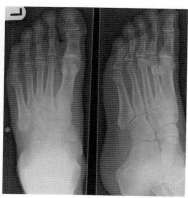

A Flexor digitorum longus

B Peroneus brevis

C Peroneus longus

D Tibialis anterior

E Tibialis posterior

17. A 40-year-old man fell from about 3m and landed on his feet. His right heel X-ray is shown in Fig. 9.5.

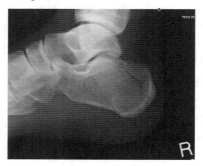

Which is the *single* most appropriate initial clinical examination? ★

A Checking the capillary filling time

B Examining for adductor magnus tendon rupture

C Examining the sensation in the foot

D Palpating the calf muscles

E Palpating the left calcaneum

18. A 45-year-old man has been having severe low back pain with radiation to his left leg for the past 12h. He has had back pain for the past few months and has received treatment with analgesics. He has altered sensation on the lateral part of the lower leg with weak extension of the left big toe. Which *single* nerve root is most likely to be affected? ★

A L2

B L3

C L4

D L5

E S1

19. A 40-year-old woman has been having severe low back pain with radiation to both legs for the past few days. She has tenderness in the low back area with muscle spasm. She has altered sensation around the anal verge and is unable to contract the anal sphincter during a digital examination. She has generally diminished reflexes in the lower limbs bilaterally. She has been given morphine IV. Which is the *single* most important initial management? ★

A Arranging a CT scan of the lumbar spine

B Arranging an X-ray of the lumbar spine

C Calling the orthopaedic senior on call urgently

D Referral to back pain clinic the next day

E Referral for urgent physiotherapy

20. A 55-year-old man has fractured his right distal radius after falling on his outstretched hand. The fracture has been reduced with a below elbow plaster cast for immobilization. He returns to the ED the next morning as the pain in his wrist has been increasing and there is pins and needles sensation in his fingers. Which is the *single* most appropriate immediate management? ★

A Admitting for elevation of the limb

B Arranging for an urgent X-ray

C Checking the radial pulse with Doppler ultrasound

D Giving IV opioid analgesia

E Splitting the cast open now

21. A 23-year-old man attends the ED after striking a glass window with his right fist. He has a laceration about 1cm long on the knuckle of the middle finger, which has now stopped bleeding. Which is the *single* most appropriate initial management? ★

A Cleaning and suturing the wound

B Discharging the patient with high arm sling

C Referral to a hand surgeon for further management

D Requesting an X-ray of the hand

E Testing for tendon damage

22. A 19-year-old man was bitten by his partner last night. He has a laceration of about 1×0.5cm on the knuckle of the right middle finger, through which the articular cartilage of the proximal end of the proximal phalanx is visible. The X-ray does not show any fracture. Which is the *single* most appropriate management? ★

A Leaving open the wound and giving antibiotics

B Primary closure with glue after cleaning

C Primary closure with Steri-Strips after irrigation

D Primary closure with sutures after cleaning

E Referral to a hand surgeon for closure after irrigation

23. A 29-year-old man sustained a laceration on the volar aspect of his right wrist while working in his garden. He is unable to bend the middle finger at the proximal interphalangeal joint with other fingers in full extension. Which is the *single* most likely tendon he has injured? ★

A Flexor digitorum profundus

B Flexor digitorum superficialis

C Flexor pollicis longus

D Palmaris longus

E Second lumbrical

24. A 27-year-old woman has a laceration on the palmer aspect of her right ring finger. She is unable to bend the terminal phalanx. Which is the *single* most likely tendon she has injured? ★

A Flexor digitorum profundus

B Flexor digitorum superficialis

C Flexor pollicis longus

D Palmaris longus

E Second lumbrical

25. A 40-year-old woman has a laceration on the dorsum of the lateral side of the wrist. She has impaired sensation on the dorsum of the first web space. Which is the *single* most likely nerve she has injured? ★

A Digital

B Dorsal cutaneous

C Medial

D Radial

E Ulnar

26. A 30-year-old man has had an accident at work (Fig. 9.6). He has been given adequate analgesia.

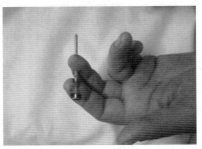

Which is the *single* most appropriate initial management? ★

A Arranging removal

B Giving antibiotics

C Giving tetanus booster

D Referral to a hand surgeon

E Sending for X-ray

27. A 30-year-old man has injured his hands in a fight (Fig. 9.7).

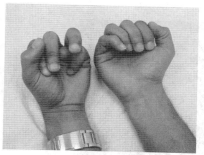

Which is the *single* most likely finger involved? ★

A Left little finger

B Left middle finger

C Left ring finger

D Right little finger

E Right ring finger

28. A 65-year-old woman fell on her outstretched left hand. The wrist is swollen and painful. Her X-ray is shown in Fig. 9.8.

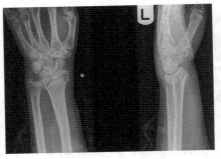

Which is the *single* most appropriate initial management? ★ ★

A Back slab after reduction

B Below elbow back slab

C Below elbow volar slab

D Broad arm sling

E Operative intervention

29. A 25-year-old nurse from a local dental clinic attends the ED in the evening following an accidental needlestick injury to her left index finger after seeing the last patient of the day. Which is the *single* most appropriate management? ★ ★ ★

A Discharging her after dressing the wound and providing reassurance

B Offering her appropriate treatment now, after assessing her in the department

C Referring her to her own GP urgently

D Referring her to the genitourinary medicine clinic on the following day

E Referring her to the occupational health department the following morning

30. A 25-year-old doctor working in a medical ward attends the ED in the evening following an accidental needlestick injury to her left index finger after bleeding a known HIV patient. Which is the *single* most appropriate immediate next step after primary assessment? ★ ★ ★

A Ask her to attend her GP for a PEP prescription

B Issue a prescription of PEP to collect from pharmacy in the morning

C Offer her PEP as soon as possible in the ED

D Withhold PEP until counselling is arranged

E Withhold PEP until the doctor's HIV status is clear

31.

A 22-year-old man bruised his finger while playing basketball and it is now swollen. The X-ray of the finger is shown in Fig. 9.9.

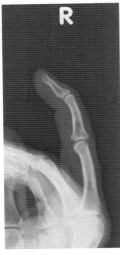

Which is the *single* most appropriate treatment? ★ ★ ★

A High arm sling

B Neighbour's strapping

C No treatment required

D Plaster of Paris immobilization

E Volar plastic splint

32. A 65-year-old woman has fallen on her outstretched right hand. She has pain around her elbow. Her X-ray is shown in Fig. 9.10.

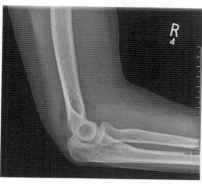

Which is the *single* most appropriate treatment? ★ ★ ★

A Back slab after reduction

B Below elbow back slab

C Collar and cuff sling

D High arm sling

E Open reduction and internal fixation

33. A 30-year-old man has had a motorbike incident and is found about 10m from his bike. He has pain and bruises around his waist. His heart rate is 80bpm, BP 110/80mmHg, and respiratory rate 20breaths/min. He has bilateral air entry to his lungs. Which is the *single* most important next management? ★ ★ ★

A Arranging a pelvic X-ray

B Examining the tip of his urethra

C Inserting a urinary catheter

D Log rolling the patient

E Performing a spring test of the pelvis

34. A 35-year-old man is found about 6m (20ft) from his car on a verge following a car accident. After being brought to the ED, he has pain around his waist. His heart rate is 82bpm, BP 112/80mmHg and respiratory rate 16breaths/min. He has bilateral air entry to his lungs and a soft non-tender abdomen. Which is the *single* most important initial management? ★ ★ ★

A Calling the general surgeons

B Giving morphine

C Performing a FAST scan

D Requesting an X-ray of the abdomen

E Requesting an X-ray of the chest

35. A 22-year-old man had a twisting injury to his knee while playing football. He says he heard a 'pop' sound at the time. The right knee immediately became swollen and painful. He could not continue to play anymore and had to be carried off the pitch in a stretcher. Which is the *single* most likely knee injury? ★ ★ ★

A Anterior cruciate ligament rupture

B Lateral collateral ligament sprain

C Medial collateral ligament sprain

D Posterior cruciate ligament rupture

E Quadriceps tendon rupture

36. A 28-year-old woman slipped on a kerb yesterday while walking and twisted her ankle, rotating the foot inwards. She has mild swelling, bruising, and tenderness distal to the lateral malleolus. She is able to weightbear. Which is the *single* most appropriate management? ★ ★ ★

A Arranging urgent physiotherapy

B Below knee back slab immobilization

C Discouraging weightbearing until fully recovered

D Double Tubigrip followed by gentle exercises

E Initial rest followed by mobilization

37. A 60-year-old woman has had severe pain in her right wrist for the past few days. She has rheumatoid arthritis with intermittent multiple joint pains. Her wrist is swollen and red, and severely painful to move. The woman has been given analgesia. Which is the *single* most appropriate diagnostic investigation? ★ ★ ★

A CRP

B Full blood count

C Joint aspiration

D No investigation required

E X-ray of the wrist

38. A 30-year-old motorcyclist has injured his right leg after colliding with a car. He has a laceration of about 3cm in length on the front of his right leg and one end of a broken tibia is protruding through the wound which otherwise looks clean. There is no neurovascular deficiency. Which *single* type of compound injury is he most likely to have? ★ ★ ★ ★

A Type I

B Type II

C Type IIIA

D Type IIIB

E Type IIIC

39. A 26-year-old man injured his right leg when he was hit by a car while crossing a road. He has a laceration about 2.5cm long in the front of the leg and a broken bone is protruding through the wound. The wound looks clean and there is no neurovascular deficiency. Which is the *single* most appropriate immediate management? ★ ★ ★ ★

A Giving analgesia

B Giving antibiotics

C Sending for an X-ray

D Taking photographs

E Taking a swab

40. A 25-year-old man injured his left leg when his motorbike collided with a tree. He has a laceration about 4cm long in the front of the leg and a piece of bone is protruding through the wound. The wound looks clean and there is no neurovascular deficiency. He has received 10mg of morphine and 2g of cefotaxime IV. Which is the *single* most appropriate next management step? ★ ★ ★ ★

A Dressing the wound after irrigation

B Giving tetanus toxoid immunoglobulin

C Sending for an X-ray of his right leg

D Taking him to theatre

E Taking swabs from the wound

41. A 55-year-old man fractured the right distal radius after falling on his outstretched hand. The fracture has been reduced with below elbow plaster cast immobilization. He returns to the ED the next morning with increasing pain in the forearm and pins and needles in his fingers. The plaster cast is removed but there is no improvement. Which is the *single* most likely diagnosis? ★ ★ ★ ★

A Compartment syndrome

B Extensor pollicis longus rupture

C Fracture fragments re-displaced

D Reflex sympathetic dystrophy syndrome

E Septic arthritis in the wrist

42. A 22-year-old woman was driving and when she slowed down to stop at a roundabout her car was hit from behind by another car. The following day she has neck pain with stiffness and tenderness in the trapezius and neck extensors on the right side. There are no other findings. Which is the *single* most important management? ★ ★ ★ ★

A Admitting for observation

B Discharging with analgesics

C Giving her a soft collar with analgesia

D Triple immobilization of neck

E X-ray of the cervical spine

43. An 85-year-old woman has had a fall. She has previously had left femoral surgery. Her pelvic X-ray is shown in Fig. 9.11.

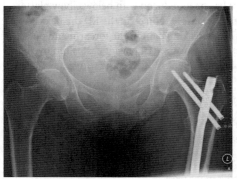

Which is the *single* most appropriate management? ★ ★ ★ ★

A Analgesia with mobilization

B CT scan of the pelvis

C Graduated skin traction

D Open reduction with manipulation

E Total hip replacement

Single Best Answers

1. E ★   OHEM, 4th edn → p416

Oozing wounds on a toe as in the patient in this scenario can be effectively closed only by suturing. Neighbour strapping is used to immobilize toes in soft tissue bruising or closed fractures. Steri-Strips will come off when they get wet due to the bleeding, but they are used for pretibial lacerations. Glue is useful in children on scalp lacerations. Its use is avoided over joints and oozing wounds. Delayed primary closure with sutures, usually 3–5 days after the injury, may be indicated when the patient presents over 6h after receiving the laceration.

2. B ★   OHEM, 4th edn → p416

Wounds more than 6h old should be closed after 3–5 days to avoid infection. The timing of closure depends on the individual wound, the patient's status, and the clinical circumstances. Primary (immediate) closure of a wound on the face can be done 24h or more after the injury. Wounds that are heavily contaminated or infected, crush injuries with significant devitalized tissue, or skin loss should not be closed immediately (primary closure). Most wounds >12h old (except clean facial wounds) may be closed 3–5 days after the injury (called delayed primary closure). Wounds that require delayed primary closure should be prepared by debridement and saline irrigation followed by packing of the wound, covered by dressing. Apply a splint if the wound is on an extremity. Prophylactic antibiotics are not required in delayed primary closure of the wounds (except human or animal bites).

Marx JA, *et al.* (eds) (2010) *Rosen's Emergency Medicine: Concepts and Clinical Practice*, 7th edn. Philadelphia: Mosby/Elsevier, pp703–4.

3. D ★   OHEM, 4th edn → pp416, 495

This is pretibial laceration, which is commonly seen following a trivial injury in an elderly person. Clean and irrigate the wound under local anaesthesia, remove any clot, and close the wound using Steri-Strips. Apply a non-adherent dressings and light compression bandage. Instruct the patient to elevate the limb whenever possible.

Arrange follow-up in 5 days' time to inspect the wound. The Steri-Strips should remain in place until the wound has healed.

As the skin in the pretibial area is very thin and friable, sutures and staples would cut through the skin and make the wound worse. Glue is not applied for the same reason. Skin grafting may be required later in some patients if the skin becomes non-viable.

4. E ★   OHEM, 4th edn → p420

The need for tetanus immunization after injury depends upon a patient's tetanus immunity status and whether the wound is 'clean' or 'tetanus prone'. In this case the wound is 'clean' and there is no need of vaccination as the patient is fully immunized. Patients may require anti-tetanus immunoglobulin with a dose of the anti-tetanus vaccine if the wound is suspected to be tetanus prone. A full course of three doses is needed in patients who have not had any prophylaxis in the past.

Tetanus-prone wounds include (please see Table 9.1 on p243):

- Wounds or burns that require surgical intervention, which has been delayed for more than 6h
- Wounds or burns that show a significant degree of devitalized tissue or a puncture-type injury, particularly where there has been contact with soil or manure
- Wounds containing foreign bodies
- Compound fractures
- Wounds or burns in patients who have systemic sepsis.

→ www.dh.gov.uk/prod_consum_dh/groups/dh_digitalassets/ documents/digitalasset/dh_122519.pdf

Immunisation against infectious disease – The Green Book (2007). Department of Health.

5. D ★   OHEM, 4th edn → p420

The need for tetanus immunization after injury depends upon a patient's tetanus status and whether the wound is 'clean' or 'tetanus-prone'. In this case, the wound is tetanus prone. Consider giving human anti-tetanus immunoglobulin (see Table 9.1 on p243).

6. C ★   OHEM, 4th edn → p424

Closure is controversial but bites on the face are preferably closed after thorough cleaning with normal saline, for cosmetic reasons. Bites cause contaminated puncture wounds that have a high risk of bacterial infection. Cat bites require prophylaxis antibiotics, as they tend to be deep puncture wounds. In cat bites, *Pasturella multocida*

Table 9.1 Department of Health immunization recommendations for clean and tetanus-prone wounds

Immunization status	Clean wound	Tetanus-prone wound	
	Vaccine	Vaccine	Human tetanus immuno-globulin
Fully immunized, i.e. has received a total of five doses of vaccine at appropriate intervals	None required	None required	Only if high risk
Primary immunization complete, boosters incomplete but up to date	None required (unless next dose due soon and convenient to give now)	None required (unless next dose due soon and convenient to give now)	Only if high risk
Primary immunization incomplete or boosters not up to date	A reinforcing dose of the vaccine and further doses as required to complete the recommended schedule (to ensure future immunity)	A reinforcing dose of the vaccine and further doses as required to complete the recommended schedule (to ensure future immunity)	Yes: one dose of human tetanus immuno-globulin in a different site
Not immunized or immunization status not known or uncertain	An immediate dose of vaccine followed by, if records confirm the need, completion of a full five-dose course to ensure future immunity	An immediate dose of vaccine followed by, if records confirm the need, completion of a full five-dose course to ensure future immunity	Yes: one dose of human tetanus immuno-globulin in a different site

Wounds, fractures, orthopaedics

is found in the infected wounds, and is sensitive to penicillin. Antibiotics prophylaxis is controversial for dog bites. *Staphylococcus* species, *Streptococcus* species, and *Bacteroides* are the causative organisms. The reported infection rate is 6–16% for patients not receiving antibiotics. Antibiotics may be considered for certain types of dog bites namely, deep puncture wounds or hand injuries or bites in the elderly population or immunocompromised patients.

Barry S, Hern HG Jr. (2010) Wound management principles. In: Marx JA, *et al.* (eds) *Rosen's Emergency Medicine: Concepts and Clinical Practice*, 7th edn. Philadelphia: Mosby/Elsevier, pp711–12.

7. D ★

Elevating the limb after applying local pressure is a safe and effective option.

A: This would not stop the bleeding and thus would not work.

B: A tourniquet should not be applied for more than 15min. Longer than this, it may compromise the vascular supply at the tip of the thumb permanently.

C: Blind application of artery forceps may damage the neurovascular bundle permanently.

E: Injection of epinephrine is contraindicated in digits as it may cause gangrene of the tip of the thumb.

8. C ★   OHEM, 4th edn → pp464–5

The patient probably has either a dislocated elbow or a displaced fracture of the elbow joint. In either situation, it is extremely important to examine the distal pulses and sensation, as the brachial artery and median artery and/or ulnar nerves may be damaged. After analgesia and X-rays the dislocation must be reduced as soon as possible under IV sedation in the ED.

A: Attempt to move an already deformed elbow would unnecessarily inflict more pain.

B: The radial nerve is not commonly injured in such a situation.

D: Examination of the shoulder is a part of the clinical assessment, which is required after the reduction of the elbow.

E: Completion of the full clinical examination (including palpating the fingers for any tenderness) may well need to wait until reduction of the elbow.

9. A ★   OHEM, 4th edn → p468

The patient has an anterior (subcoracoid) dislocation of the left shoulder joint. The most commonly involved nerve in such injuries is the axillary nerve (5–54% incidence), which winds round the surgical neck of the humerus. This injury is more frequent in patients aged >50 years. It is detected by testing for loss of sensation over the lateral aspect of the shoulder (the 'badge' area) supplied by the axillary nerve. The motor function is assessed by asking the patient to attempt abduction and feeling the contraction of deltoid muscle, which cannot be reliably assessed until some weeks after the dislocation has been reduced. However, the motor function is more accurate than the sensory testing. The brachial plexus and radial nerve may also be damaged in such injuries.

Daya M, Nakamura Y. (2010) Shoulder. In: Marx JA, *et al.* (eds) *Rosen's Emergency Medicine: Concepts and Clinical Practice*, 7th edn. Philadelphia: Mosby/Elsevier, p579.

10. A ★   OHEM, 4th edn → p482

The patient has a posterior dislocation of the left hip prosthesis – the typical deformity that occurs in such a situation. The sciatic nerve damage must be checked by examining dorsiflexion of the foot and sensation below the knee. Extension of the knee is achieved by contraction of the quadriceps, which are supplied by the femoral nerve (L2–L4). Flexion of the hip joint is primarily by the iliopsoas muscles, which are supplied by the femoral nerve (L2–L4) and lumbar plexus (L1–L5). The sensation is carried by the genitofemoral nerve (L1) from the area of the femoral triangle. The lateral surface of the thigh is supplied by the lateral cutaneous femoral nerve (L2, L3). None of the other four options is relevant to the posterior dislocation of the hip joint.

→ www.instantanatomy.net/leg/nerves/cutaneoussupplygeneral.html

11. B ★   OHEM, 4th edn → p482

The patient has had an injury to her right hip, a common occurrence in elderly woman, even after a trivial fall. The priority is to give analgesia within 20min. An X-ray should be arranged within an hour. Referral to orthopaedics is done once the X-ray has confirmed a fracture. Social services may be involved if there is no fracture, the pain is under control, and the patient does not require in-hospital treatment for any acute medical condition. Traction is not an option in this situation.

12. D ★   OHEM, 4th edn → pp489, 492

In injuries to the medial collateral ligament of the knee, the valgus stress test may be positive. This is done by gently applying a valgus stress to the knee joint (moving the lower leg laterally) keeping the knee in 0° and 30° flexion. Examine for laxity or pain and this must be compared with the other side. Isolated collateral ligament tears are detected only with the knee in slight flexion because in extension, the cruciate ligaments and capsule provide considerable stability. Laxity in full extension denotes complete collateral ligament tear with injury to the cruciate ligaments or other structures.

A: The anterior draw test is done to check the anterior cruciate ligament injury. To do this test bring the knee to 90° flexion, sit on the patient's foot and hold the leg with both hands around the upper tibia. Ensure the quadriceps and hamstrings muscles are relaxed. Using the clinician's body weight, gently rock backwards and forwards looking for anterior glide (draw) of the tibia (indicating rupture of the anterior cruciate ligament) or posterior glide of the tibia (indicating rupture of the posterior cruciate ligament). For the anterior draw test to be positive, the medial meniscus or meniscotibial ligament must also be damaged. Positive findings with an anterior drawer test is conclusive evidence of an anterior cruciate ligament tear, but not every such tear will show positive findings on the anterior drawer test.

B: A patellar tap test is done to diagnose presence of fluid in the knee (knee effusion).

C: Ask the patient to straight leg raise. The ability to do this against resistance virtually excludes the quadriceps or patellar tendon rupture.

E: The varus test is done by moving the lower leg medially, which tests the lateral collateral ligament complex.

Perform these tests on each knee and compare both sides.

→ www.maitrise-orthop.com/corpusmaitri/orthopaedic/mo56_knee_joint/knee_joint.shtml

13. D ★   OHEM, 4th edn → p494

The common peroneal nerve may be damaged in proximal fibular injuries. The injury to the nerve causes weakness of dorsiflexion of the ankle and reduced sensation on the lateral aspect of the forefoot. Plantar flexion of the toes and foot are mediated by the tibial nerve.

14. D ★   OHEM, 4th edn → pp500–1

The dorsalis pedis artery pulse must be checked immediately in this dislocated (deformed) ankle. The artery may be damaged in such situations, resulting in compromised blood supply of the foot. The colour of the foot may be deceptive if the patient has been in the cold outside. The other clinical tests may be done later.

15. A ★   OHEM, 4th edn → p502

Inversion of the foot (when the sole of the foot turns to face medially as the ankle is planterflexed) causes damage to the structures around the lateral malleolus, most commonly the anterior talofibular ligament (Fig. 9.12). Almost two-thirds of ankle sprains are anterior talofibular injuries. If the force is significant, the next ligament to be involved is the calcaneofibular ligament. Deltoid ligaments situated on the medial side are injured when there is an external force, i.e. with eversion injuries. Inferior talofibular and transverse ligaments are rarely involved in inversion injuries.

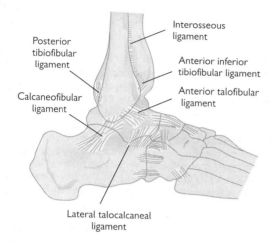

Interosseous ligament

Posterior tibiofibular ligament

Anterior inferior tibiofibular ligament

Calcaneofibular ligament

Anterior talofibular ligament

Lateral talocalcaneal ligament

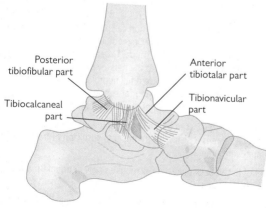

Posterior tibiofibular part

Anterior tibiotalar part

Tibiocalcaneal part

Tibionavicular part

16. B ★   OHEM, 4th edn → p505

Fig. 9.4 in the question shows fracture at the base of the fifth metatarsal. Following an inversion injury to the ankle, an avulsion fracture of the base of the fifth metatarsal is caused by the pull of the peroneus brevis tendon, which is attached at the base. The other options are not involved in this injury.

17. E ★   OHEM, 4th edn → p504

Calcaneal fractures most often follow a fall from height directly onto the heels. Always exclude associated injuries of the cervical and lumbar spine, pelvis, hips, or knees. Such fractures are commonly bilateral, so, examine both calcanei. Also examine the Achilles tendon for injury and request specific calcaneal X-rays.

18. D ★   OHEM, 4th edn → pp508-9

The patient has L5 nerve root compression. The L5 nerve root supplies sensation to the lower lateral part of the leg and great toe, and power to extensor hallucis longus. The L2 root is responsible for sensation on the front and medial side of the middle third of the thigh and flexion of the hip (iliopsoas). L3 supplies sensation to the front of the knee and together with L4 extends the knee. L4 covers sensation of the medial lower leg and provides motor supply to the quadriceps (covers knee jerk). S1 covers sensation of the little toe and lateral foot, power to foot plantar flexors, and the ankle jerk. Fig. 9.13 overleaf shows the front and back dermatomes.

19. C ★   OHEM, 4th edn → p509

The patient has cauda equina syndrome (bilateral pain with altered sensation in the perianal area with reduced/ loss of anal sphincter tone). This is an orthopaedic emergency and requires immediate attention of the orthopaedics senior on call. An urgent MRI scan may be arranged if available followed by immediate surgery for mechanical decompression of the cauda. Urgent decompression may limit the symptoms and damage to the nerves. Therefore, every patient with back pain should have a full neurological examination of the lower limbs including checking for sensation around perineum/perianal area and tone of the anal sphincter.

A and B: X-ray and CT scan of the lumber spine are done in an emergency if there is a history of trauma and suspicion of fracture of the lumbar vertebrae.

D: Referral to the back pain clinic is required only in traumatic stable fractures of the lumbar spine.

E: Urgent physiotherapy is sometimes required in simple back pain which has not improved much after regular analgesic medication.

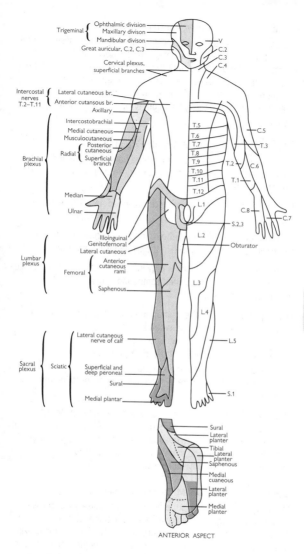

Trigeminal {
Ophthalmic division
Maxillary divison
Mandibular divison
Great auricular, C.2, C.3
Cervical plexus,
superficial branches

V
C.2
C.3
C.4

Intercostal nerves T.2–T.11 {
Lateral cutaneous br.
Anterior cutaneous br.
Axillary

Brachial plexus {
Intercostobrachial
Medial cutaneous
Musculocutaneous
Radial {
Posterior cutaneous
Superficial branch
Median
Ulnar

T.5
T.6
T.7
T.8
T.9
T.10
T.11
T.12

C.5
T.3
T.2
C.6
T.1
C.8
C.7

Lumbar plexus {
Illoinguinal
Genitofemoral
Lateral cutaneous
Femoral {
Anterior cutaneous rami
Saphenous

L.1
S.2,3
L.2
Obturator
L.3
L.4
L.5

Sacral plexus { Sciatic {
Lateral cutaneous nerve of calf
Superficial and deep peroneal
Sural
Medial plantar

S.1

Sural
Lateral planter
Tibial
Lateral planter
Saphenous
Medial cuaneous
Lateral planter
Medial planter

ANTERIOR ASPECT

249

20. E ★ OHEM, 4th edn → p436

The patient has features of suspected vascular compromise from the cast application. So you need to act immediately: cut the wool and bandages of the back slab until the skin is visible along the whole length of the limb. Assess the neurovascular status of the limb. Elevation will not help much, an X-ray in unnecessary and radial artery involvement is a very late sign. IV opioids will not relieve such pain.

21. E ★ OHEM, 4th edn → pp442–7

It is extremely important to examine the hand for damage to the extensor tendons as it would have significant implications on the next step of management.

A: Closure of the wound is not recommended until a glass foreign body is excluded by X-ray.

B: Discharging the patient without adequate clinical examination and exclusion of a glass piece in the wound is inappropriate.

C: Referral to hand surgeons is only indicated if there is an evidence of tendon damage or suspected compound injury to the metacarpophalangeal joint.

D: X-ray of the hand is the next appropriate step to rule out any glass foreign body inside the wound.

22. E ★ OHEM, 4th edn → pp 424–6

This is a compound injury to the metacarpophalangeal joint that needs irrigation and closure by a hand surgeon. The other options are inappropriate.

Bites (both human and animal) cause contaminated puncture wounds, contaminated crush injuries, or both. All carry a high risk of bacterial infection. Explore fresh bite wounds under appropriate anaesthesia, and debride and clean thoroughly. Prophylactic antibiotics should be advisable in such cases.

23. B ★ OHEM, 4th edn → pp444–5

Injury to flexor digitorum superficialis tendon causes weakness of flexion of the finger at the proximal interphalangeal joint. The superficial flexor tendons bifurcate near the base of the proximal phalanges and surround the tendons of flexor digitorum profundus before inserting on the middle phalanges of digits II–V. The flexor digitorum profundus lies deep to the flexor digitorum superficialis at this level. It flexes the distal interphalangeal joint and all joints flexed by flexor digitorum superficialis. The flexor digitorum superficialis is tested individually by asking the patient to flex the proximal interphalangeal joint while the other fingers are held in extension to block the flexion produced by the flexor digitorum profundus.

The above clinical examination should be performed in every hand injury case to test the integrity of the superficialis tendon along side others.

Lyn ET, Mailhot T. (2010) Hand. In: Marx JA, *et al.* (eds) *Rosen's Emergency Medicine: Concepts and Clinical Practice*, 7th edn. Philadelphia: Mosby/Elsevier, pp495–6.

24. A ★ OHEM, 4th edn → pp444–5

Injury to the flexor digitorum profundus tendon causes weakness of flexion of the finger at the distal interphalangeal joint. The tendons insert at the base of the distal phalanx and act primarily to flex the distal interphalangeal joint. They are more commonly injured in finger lacerations because of their paradoxical superficial position.

This is a common clinical examination which should be performed in every hand injury case to test the profundus tendon along side others.

Lyn ET, Mailhot T. (2010) Hand. In: Marx JA, *et al.* (eds) *Rosen's Emergency Medicine: Concepts and Clinical Practice*, 7th edn. Philadelphia: Mosby/Elsevier, pp495–6.

25. D ★ OHEM, 4th edn → p444

The dorsum of the first web space is exclusively supplied by the cutaneous branch of the radial nerve. The digital nerves supply the fingers, medial to the lateral three and half fingers on the palmar side and the medial one and a half of the fingers by the ulnar nerve.

26. E ★ OHEM, 4th edn → p415

The nail fired from a nail gun has pierced through the pulps of the index and middle fingers. After giving analgesia, the next step would be to send for X-rays before attempting removal or referring to a hand surgeon as this would depend on the X-ray results and local policy. Antibiotics should be given after removal of the foreign body and thorough irrigation of the wound.

27. C ★ OHEM, 4th edn → pp444–5

To test for the rotational deformity of a finger, the patient is asked to gently flex all his fingers. The tip of the fingers should grossly point towards the centre of the distal crease of the wrist. In this case, the left ring finger is significantly rotated, which is a diagnosis made by inspection of the flexed finger and should not to be missed. It is caused by a spiral fracture of the shaft of the metacarpal of the finger. The other fingers are normal. Such cases should be initially treated by analgesia, elevation, and referral to a hand surgeon after taking X-rays; they may require internal fixation.

28. A ★ ★   OHEM, 4th edn → pp458–9

This is Colles' fracture, which affects the distal radius within 2.5cm of the wrist. The distal fragment is angulated to point dorsally, giving the characteristic clinical dinner fork deformity. This fracture is displaced significantly and requires manipulation under local anaesthesia followed by immobilization by a below elbow back slab. A simple broad arm sling or volar back slab is not the appropriate treatment. Such patients should be referred to a fracture clinic for follow-up after satisfactory reduction and immobilization. The patient may require operative reduction if the fragment slips again.

29. B ★ ★ ★   OHEM, 4th edn → p428

This is an emergency. The wound must be immediately washed with soap and water. The patient would require full clinical evaluation and risk assessment for possible PEP for HIV as soon as possible, preferably within an hour of the injury. Enquire about the patient who was being treated when the nurse had the injury, and particularly whether they were known to be high risk. A detailed history of the needlestick injury should be taken, particularly exploring how much blood from the needle she might have been exposed to. Discuss the risk assessment with your senior to help decide whether to give PEP. Ensure that the nurse is already immunized against hepatitis B. If PEP is given, the nurse should be followed up in the genitourinary clinic. She should inform her own occupational health department about the incident as soon as possible. Such patients should not referred to GPs as the GPs may not have provision of offering PEP and valuable treatment time would be wasted.

→ www.advisorybodies.doh.gov.uk/eaga/publications.htm

30. C ★ ★ ★   OHEM, 4th edn → p428

This is an emergency. The wound must be immediately washed with soap and water. The recipient would require full assessment followed by PEP as soon as possible, preferably within an hour of the injury if the source patient (donor) is known to be or suspected of being HIV positive. The drugs are most effective if started within an hour of exposure. Ensure that the recipient is already immunized against hepatitis B. If PEP is given, they should be followed up in the genitourinary clinic. The doctor (recipient's) should inform the occupational health department about the incident the next working day. These patients should not be referred to GPs as the GPs may not have provision of offering PEP and valuable treatment time would be wasted. There is no need to check the HIV status as the doctor is already working on the wards carrying out invasive procedures (taking blood samples in this situation). The pharmacy would be closed in the evening and sending the patient to pharmacy would lose valuable time. The ED should give the first dose of medication straightwary after briefly counselling her.

→ www.advisorybodies.doh.gov.uk/eaga/publications.htm

31. E ★ ★ ★   OHEM, 4th edn → p448

This is a common extensor tendon injury, which occurs when the tendon ruptures near its distal attachment at the base of the distal phalanx. This may or may not be associated with a fracture of the base of the distal phalanx. The distal phalanx develops a flexion position and an inability to extend it called extension lag.

Such injuries, called 'Mallet finger deformity' must be treated in a volar or dorsal plastic splint to keep the distal interphalangeal joint continuously in extension for at least six weeks. If the injury is open or the fracture involving more than a third of the joint surface, it may require operative treatment. A high arm sling may be given to help reduce pain and swelling after the splint. Neighbour's strapping (immobilizing the finger after strapping with the neighbouring finger with a tape) or plaster of Paris immobilization is not the correct treatment in this case.

32. C ★ ★ ★   OHEM, 4th edn → p464

The patient has elevated anterior and posterior fat pad signs (the dark triangular area elevated from the anterior and posterior supracondylar area in Fig. 9.10), signifying an effusion inside the joint. Always assume that a radial head/neck fracture is present. Provide analgesia, a collar and cuff sling and arrange a review to ensure that full movement is regained.

33. B ★ ★ ★   OHEM, 4th edn → pp480–1

This patient has had a high-speed injury as he has been thrown a few metres away from his motorbike. On initial examination during the primary survey, it is important to inspect the pelvic area and see if there is bruising around the pelvis or an open wound. Do not attempt the spring test as it is unreliable, unnecessary and, may cause increased bleeding. On inspection of the urethra a drop of blood at the meatus may signify urethral injury.

A urinary catheter should not be inserted in such situation. The mechanism of injury makes it likely that he may have a pelvic fracture, so log rolling may wait until later when a pelvic X-ray has excluded an unstable pelvic fracture. Inspection of the urethral tip for blood is important to aid further decision making, including the need for a pelvic X-ray.

34. B ★ ★ ★ OHEM, 4th edn → pp328–9

This patient has had a high-speed injury in which he has been thrown a few metres away from his car, possibly ejected. On initial examination during primary survey, it is important to examine the ABCDE. These parameters are within normal limits in this patient. The next most important step is to address the patient's pain. X-rays of the pelvis and other parts of the body may wait until he is stabilized. A FAST scan may be performed but there is no indication of any abdominal injury, so it can wait. There is no indication to take him to the theatre. Performing the abdominal film is useless in the ED.

35. A ★ ★ ★ OHEM, 4th edn → p492

The cruciate ligaments are the primary stabilizers for the anterior and posterior displacement of the tibia on the femur. Anterior cruciate ligament injuries are more common than posterior cruciate ligament injuries. The former injuries particularly occur during football, skiing, and vehicular collisions, when the knee is twisted in a flexed position, keeping the foot fixed to the ground. Immediate pain and swelling (because of haemarthrosis), inability to weightbear and a history of an audible 'pop' are all suggestive of an anterior cruciate ligament tear. The diagnosis can often be made from the history alone. Posterior cruciate ligament injuries occur following a direct blow from the front to the knee in a flexed position (dashboard injury in vehicular collisions). It is unusual to have an injury to the posterior cruciate ligament in sporting activities. The injury mentioned in the scenario may be associated with medial collateral ligament rupture. In an isolated sprain of the medial collateral ligament, the bruise is localized on the medial side of the knee and is not associated with immediate swelling in the knee. Lateral collateral ligament injuries occur due to a direct blow from the lateral direction in a hyperextended knee and are usually not associated with immediate swelling. Rupture of the quadriceps tendon may occur from a sudden violent contraction of the quadriceps muscle or from a direct injury. There is no knee swelling in the early stages.

Fig. 9.14 shows the cruciate and collateral ligaments: (a) posterior view of the right knee in extension, and (b) anterior view of the right knee in flexion.

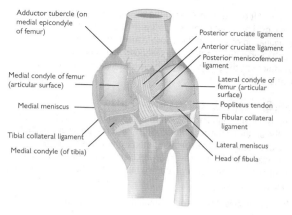

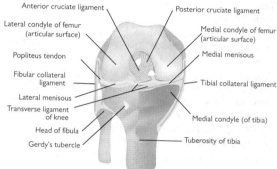

36. E ★ ★ ★   OHEM, 4th edn → p502

Advise patients to rest initially for a couple of days with the ankle elevated above the hip level and application of ice (bags of frozen peas applied four times a day for a couple of days). As soon as the symptoms allow, the patient should start gentle exercise and begin weightbearing. Some serious injuries when the patient is unable to weightbear may require treatment by back slab immobilization followed by physiotherapy. Double Tubigrip has been proven to be of no value.

37. C ★ ★ ★   OHEM, 4th edn → pp510–1

The patient possibly has septic arthritis, which has an increased incidence among patients with rheumatoid arthritis, those taking steroids, the immunosuppressed and at the extremes of age. In septic arthritis typically one joint is affected. Although full blood count, ESR or CRP, and X-ray of the wrist are useful investigations, the most important diagnostic test is joint aspiration and examination of synovial fluid. Such patients must not be discharged without a definitive diagnosis and appropriate treatment as the sepsis may progress to complete joint destruction within 24h.

38. B ★ ★ ★ ★ OHEM, 4th edn → p420

This is a compound fracture, which occurs when the fracture is open to the air through a skin wound. Such fractures are all at very high risk of infection and can be associated with gross soft tissue damage, severe haemorrhage, or vascular injury. They are treated as an orthopaedic emergency requiring rapid assessment and treatment to prevent osteomyelitis.

The Gustilo classification of compound injuries is as follows:

- Type I: Compound fracture where the wound is <1cm and appears clean.
- Type II: Compound fracture where the wound is >1cm but not associated with extensive soft tissue damage, tissue loss, or flap laceration.
- Type IIIA: Either a compound fracture with adequate soft tissue coverage of bone despite extensive soft tissue damage or flap laceration of any fracture involving high energy trauma or bone shattering regardless of wound size.
- Type IIIB: Compound fracture with extensive soft tissue loss with periosteal stripping and exposure of bone.
- Type IIIC: Compound fracture associated with vascular injury needing repair.

Gustilo RB, Anderson JB. (1976) Prevention of infection in the treatment of one thousand and twenty-five open fractures of long bones: retrospective and prospective analyses. *J Bone Joint Surg Am* **58**(4):453–8.

39. A ★ ★ ★ ★ OHEM, 4th edn → p420

Arrange for analgesia first, as the others steps may take longer or may be done later. An antibiotic is important but can wait until after analgesia is given. To avoid repeated exposure and thus infection owing to inspection of the wound by different specialists, a photograph may be taken just before wound management, which is done after giving analgesia. A swab is no longer recommended. X-rays should be done once the wound is cleaned and dressed, and the limb is immobilized.

40. A ★ ★ ★ ★ OHEM, 4th edn → pp432–3

After irrigating the wound with normal saline, cover with a sterile moist dressing. Immobilize the limb in a POP back slab. Do not inspect the wound repeatedly as this greatly increases the risk of wound infection.

B: Tetanus immunoglobulin may be given once the wound management is complete.

C: X-rays should be done once the wound is cleaned and dressed, and the limb immobilized.

D: Prior taking the patient to theatre, provide adequate fluid replacement (if indicated), analgesia, splintage, antibiotics, and tetanus prophylaxis. These steps could be completed while the orthopaedics senior doctor is contacted.

E: Taking swabs for culture and sensitivity from the wound at this stage is not recommended as they do not alter management and are poor predictors of deep infection.

41. A ★ ★ ★ ★ OHEM, 4th edn → pp408, 436

This man has compartment syndrome caused by damage to the muscles entrapped within their compartment, which results in an increase in the compartmental pressure. Subsequently this obstructs muscular blood flow, resulting in ischaemia and oedema of the muscles, which results in further increase in the pressure causing muscle death. The muscle pain, swelling of part of the limb, and tenderness may not be present at the time of presentation or immediately after the injury.

B: Extensor pollicis longus tendon rupture typically occurs a few weeks after the reduction and does not cause the symptoms described in the scenario.

C: Displacement of a fracture fragment may occur if the plaster cast is not applied correctly, but it would not cause the above symptoms as described.

D: Reflex sympathetic dystrophy syndrome (Sudek's osteodystrophy) (http://tra.sagepub.com/cgi/reprint/9/3/151) can occur after even a trivial sprain or laceration on the hand. The actual reason is unknown, but it is believed to be due to overactivity of the sympathetic nervous system following a stimulus. The symptoms are burning sensation in the hand and skin changes.

E: The likelihood of septic arthritis in such a situation is minimal. The symptoms would be localized redness and swelling in the joint.

42. B ★★★★ OHEM, 4th edn → p476

This patient has been involved in a low impact incident and has typically developed pain and stiffness after a certain amount of time. The diagnosis is a soft tissue injury to the neck ('whiplash' type injury). This patient does not require X-rays or a CT scan. Appropriate analgesia and regular gentle exercise should help her. Encourage early movements. She may be referred for physiotherapy if her situation does not improve within a week. Triple immobilization (immobilization of the head and neck with semi-rigid collar, head blocks, and adhesive tapes) is done when there is a suspicion of cervical spine injury.

43. A ★★★★

This patient has a left-sided superior pubic ramus fracture, which is common in elderly people but often missed, particularly when the focus is on a potential fractured neck of femur). Refer to orthopaedics for analgesia and initial bed rest followed by mobilization.

B: CT scan of the pelvis is required if a patient has trauma resulting from a significant force (e.g. vehicular collision).

C: Skin traction used to be a form of management of fractured neck of femur, before the introduction of prostheses.

D: Open reduction and manipulation is required if there is dislocation of a joint and failed closed reduction.

E: Total hip replacement is done for subcapital fracture of neck of femur in younger, active patients in whom a hemiarthroplasty is inappropriate or in severe osteoarthritis.

CHAPTER 10
SURGERY

'The patient is the centre of the medical universe around which all our works revolve and towards which all our efforts trend.'

JB Murphy

Among surgical patients presenting to the ED, abdominal pain is the most common complaint, comprising 10% of ED visits. Evaluation of such patients in the ED is often challenging for a variety of reasons, such as the variability in the description of the perception of pain in individual patients, variable and changing physical findings with time, and life-threatening conditions presenting as seemingly benign symptoms.

I always advise inexperienced doctors working in the ED to bear in mind seven *time bombs* that may be 'sitting inside' every adult patient's abdomen who presents with abdominal pain. Patients who are discharged, but in whom one of these diagnoses was missed, will be blue-lighted back to the department dead. Therefore, before discharging a patient presenting with acute abdomen pain, all such conditions as listed below must be excluded beyond reasonable doubt. These conditions are:

- Ruptured AAA
- Hollow viscus perforation
- Mesenteric ischaemia
- Ruptured ectopic pregnancy
- Acute pancreatitis
- Intestinal obstruction
- Acute myocardial infarction.

Acute (inferior) myocardial infarction may present as upper abdominal pain and cannot afford to be missed. Patients >50 years presenting with abdominal pain must have an ECG in the ED, not only for detecting acute myocardial infarction, but for other associated cardiac problems precipitating an abdominal catastrophe.

Elderly patients are more likely to have life-threatening conditions such as a ruptured AAA, mesenteric ischaemia, peptic perforation, and diverticulitis. Atypical presentations and rapid progression of these diseases, coupled with decreased diagnostic accuracy, may increase the risk of mortality in elderly patients. The only way to avoid the above is, as importantly as in other parts of medicine, by taking an accurate history, performing a thorough full clinical examination, arranging appropriate investigations rapidly, and making the correct decisions as to whether or not urgent surgery is required. Even with advanced imaging techniques, a good understanding of background clinical information is of utmost importance for accurate interpretation of imaging findings.

This chapter includes questions on acute abdominal emergencies to give the reader an insight into the latest management strategies for these situations. ■

SINGLE BEST ANSWERS

1. A 62-year-old man has had a gradual onset of pain in his abdomen over the past few days. The pain was initially colicky but now has become constant. He has vomited several times, feels bloated, and cannot remember when he last opened his bowels. His temperature is 36.8°C, heart rate 106bpm, BP 120/80mmHg, and respiratory rate 20 breaths/min. He has distension and generalized tenderness in the abdomen. He has been given analgesia and his X-ray is shown in Fig. 10.1.

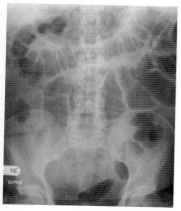

Which is the *single* most appropriate next step in management? ★

A Arranging for erect chest and repeat abdominal plain film

B Arranging urgent ultrasonography in the ED

C Discharging after arranging routine outpatient surgical referral

D Giving enema and an antiemetic followed by discharge with laxatives

E Starting IV crystalloids and inserting nasogastric tube

2. A 20-year-old woman has been having severe pain in her back passage while opening her bowels for the past few days. She also noticed some fresh blood on the toilet paper. This has happened before, but improved on its own. She has a skin tag in the 6 o'clock position. Further anal examination is not possible because of pain. She has been given analgesia. Which is the *single* most effective management? ★

A Anal dilators

B Digital anal stretching under GA

C High-fibre diet with laxatives

D Injection of phenol in arachis oil

E Referral to a surgeon

3. A 70-year-old man suddenly developed severe pain in the lower part of his abdomen. He is unable to pass water and is distressed. On examination, the lower part of his abdomen is distended, tender, and dull on percussion. Which is the *single* most appropriate initial management? ★

A Arranging abdominal X-ray

B Giving IV morphine

C Inserting a urinary catheter

D Sending blood for amylase

E Starting IV fluids

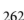

4. A 22-year-old man has a sudden onset of severe pain in the right groin and lower abdomen. He has vomited once. The right scrotum is red, swollen and tender. His urine results are: white cells –ve, nitrites –ve, protein +ve. Which is the *single* most likely diagnosis? ★

A Acute epididymoorchitis

B Scrotal cellulitis

C Strangulated hernia

D Testicular torsion

E Ureteric colic

5. A 28-year-old woman who is breastfeeding has pain in her left breast. The outer upper quadrant of the left breast is red, swollen, and tender. Which is the *single* most likely causative organism? ★

A *Staphylococcus aureus*

B *Staphylococcus epidermidis*

C *Streptococcus faecalis*

D *Streptococcus pyogenes*

E *Streptococcus viridans*

6. A 78-year-old man suddenly developed pain in his back. He is feeling dizzy and unwell and is sweaty and pale. The pain is constant and radiating to the left groin. His pulse is 100bpm and BP 100/80mmHg. He does not have any neurological signs in his lower limbs. Which is the *single* most appropriate management? ★

A Arranging abdominal ultrasound scan

B Arranging spinal X-rays

C Arranging X-ray of kidney, urinary bladder

D Giving diclofenac rectally

E Referral to the orthopaedic surgeon

7. A 50-year-old man with long-standing alcohol misuse has been vomiting and has had severe pain in the upper part of his abdomen for a couple of hours. The pain is radiating to the back and he is distressed and sweaty. His heart rate is 120bpm, BP 100/60mmHg, and respiratory rate 28 breaths/min. He has tenderness and severe pain on percussion in the epigastrium. Which is the *single* most likely biochemistry result? ★ ★ ★

A Na⁺ 120mmol/L; K⁺ 3.9mmol/L; Creatinine 76μmol/L; Urea 5.7mmol/L; Calcium ²⁺ 2.14mmol/L; Phosphate 1.0mmol/L

B Na⁺ 130mmol/L; K⁺4.0mmol/L; Creatinine 80μmol/L; Urea 5.9mmol/L; Calcium ²⁺ 2.04mmol/L; Phosphate 1.3mmol/L

C Na⁺ 136mmol/L; K⁺ 4.1mmol/L; Creatinine 85μmol/L; Urea 5.9mmol/L; Calcium ²⁺ 2.65mmol/L; Phosphate 0.8mmol/L

D Na⁺ 140mmol/L; K⁺ 4.1mmol/L; Creatinine 99μmol/L; Urea 7.9mmol/L; Calcium ²⁺ 1.14mmol/L; Phosphate 1.0mmol/L

E Na⁺ 144mmol/L; K⁺ 5.2mmol/L; Creatinine 110μmol/L; Urea 9.9mmol/L; Calcium ²⁺ 3.12mmol/L; Phosphate 1.3mmol/L

8. An 82-year-old man who has had varicose veins in both lower limbs for many years, has started bleeding from just above the right ankle after catching his leg on a piece of furniture. His pulse is 70bpm and BP 140/80mmHg. There is brisk bleeding from a tuft of venules just above the right medial malleolus. Which is the *single* most appropriate immediate management? ★ ★ ★

A Applying an adrenaline (epinephrine)-soaked gauze

B Applying a pressure bandage followed by elevation

C Arranging immediate cauterization

D Arranging injection sclerotherapy

E Arranging percutaneous vascular embolisation

9. A 28-year-old man has been having severe pain in the abdomen and vomiting for the last couple of hours. His pulse is 120bpm and BP 110/80mmHg. He has a very tender lump in the right groin just above and medial to the inguinal ligament, which has no cough impulse. Which is the *single* most appropriate immediate management? ★ ★ ★

A Admitting him on the surgical ward – only if the abdominal X-ray is abnormal

B Arranging surgical outpatient referral after giving him a truss

C Discharging home after successful forced reduction

D Discharging once the pain is reduced after giving him analgesia

E Referral to the surgeons for urgent operation after giving him analgesia

10. An 82-year-old woman has had pain in her abdomen for the past week and has been opening her bowels irregularly. She has vomited once and feels bloated. Her X-ray is shown in Fig. 10.2.

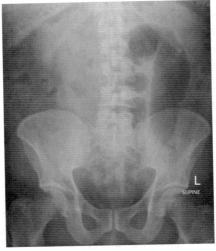

Which is the *single* most likely diagnosis? ★ ★ ★

A Caecal volvulus

B Gall stone ileus

C Left obstructed femoral hernia

D Sigmoid volvulus

E Small intestinal volvulus

11. A 72-year-old man is brought in to the ED as he has not been able to pass urine for 4h. He is in severe pain. The lower abdomen is distended, tender, and dull on percussion. While trying to catheterize him, the doctor meets slight resistance after introducing the catheter about 5cm. Which is the *single* most appropriate management? ★ ★ ★

A Applying force to push the catheter down the urethra

B Inserting a suprapubic catheter instead

C Referral to urology on-call team for completing the catheterization

D Repositioning the penis in between the patient's legs and trying again

E Trying inserting with the help of a catheter introducer

12. A 52-year-old previously healthy woman has suddenly developed colicky pain in her upper and mid abdomen. She has vomited once. Her temperature is 36.8°C, heart rate 100bpm, BP 150/90mmHg, and respiratory rate 20 breaths/min. She has tenderness in the right upper abdominal area. Her WBC is 10×10^9/L, CRP 20mg/L, albumin 40gm/L, ALP 260IU/L, AST 30IU/L, bilirubin 15μmol/L, and γ-glutamyl transpeptidase 30IU/L. The pain is better and the abdominal examination is unremarkable after analgesia. Which is the *single* most appropriate management? ★ ★ ★

A Admitting to the surgical ward for further investigation

B Admitting to the surgical ward for IV antibiotics

C Arranging an urgent CT scan in the ED

D Discharging the patient with oral antibiotics followed by ultrasonography

E Follow-up by GP for reassessment followed by ultrasonography

EXTENDED MATCHING QUESTIONS

Diagnosis of acute abdominal pain

For each of the following scenarios, choose the most likely diagnosis from the list of options below.
Each answer may be used once, more than once, or not at all.

A Acute appendicitis

B Acute cholecystitis

C Acute diverticulitis

D Acute myocardial infarction

E Acute pancreatitis

F Intestinal obstruction

G Mesenteric infarction

H Peptic perforation

I Ruptured AAA

J Sigmoid volvulus

K Ureteric colic

1. A 29-year-old man has been having pain in his central abdomen since yesterday and he started vomiting last night. The stabbing pain radiates to his right lower abdomen. His temperature is 37.4°C, pulse rate 74bpm, BP 148/100mmHg, and respiratory rate 14 breaths/min. He has tenderness in his right lower abdomen with peritonism.

2. A 50-year-old man has had sharp and constant pain in the upper part of his abdomen for 2 days. The pain is now worse and radiating to the back. He had a cholecystectomy 5 years ago for stones. He is distressed and sweaty and has started vomiting. His heart rate is 100bpm, BP 110/60mmHg, and respiratory rate 24 breaths/min. He has tenderness and severe pain on percussion in the epigastrium. The lower abdomen is soft and non-tender.

3. A 72-year-old woman has developed sudden pain in her upper abdomen. She previously had abdominal discomfort for a while. She has hypertension, hyperlipidaemia, rheumatoid arthritis, and angina. Her heart rate is 100bpm, BP 150/90mmHg, and respiratory rate 24 breaths/min. She has generalized tenderness and pain on percussion in the abdomen. The bowel sounds are absent. The ECG shows a heart rate of 104/min.

4. A 78-year-old woman has suddenly developed severe pain in the whole abdomen. She is on aspirin, digoxin, simvastatin, and atenolol. Her heart rate is irregular at 120bpm, BP 110/80mmHg, and respiratory rate 26 breaths/min. The abdomen is slightly distended and diffusely minimally tender.

5. A 67-year-old man has had constant pain in the left lower abdomen for the past few days. His temperature is 37.9°C, heart rate 90bpm, BP 140/85mmHg, and respiratory rate 20 breaths/min. He is tender in the lower left part of the abdomen.

Single Best Answers

1. E ★   OHEM, 4th edn → p528

The history and the abdominal film are suggestive of intestinal obstruction. The abdominal film (Fig. 10.1) shows distended loops of small bowel. The patient requires IV crystalloid, nasogastric tube insertion, oxygen, an antiemetic, and urgent referral to the surgical on-call team.

B: Outpatient referral is an inappropriate action.

C: Ultrasonography may be difficult to interpret because of loops of bowel full of gas. Also it may not be helpful in this situation. An erect chest X-ray should have been done with this supine abdominal film but an erect abdominal film is not indicated.

Option D may be fatal in such a situation.

2. C ★   OHEM, 4th edn → p534

The patient has a typical history of an anal fissure, often associated with constipation. The addition of fibre to the diet, use of stool softeners and adequate water intake, are simple and helpful measures. Warm baths and topical anaesthetic agents will help relieve the pain. Anal dilators are usually associated with low compliance, therefore are of little benefit. Anal stretching is no longer popular because of the risk of developing anal incontinence, and because of the requirement of GA, it is not an option in the ED. Injection of phenol in arachis oil is a treatment for haemorrhoids, not anal fissure. As almost all acute fissures should heal with conservative management, referral to a surgeon is unnecessary.

Williams NS, Bulstrode CJK, O'Connell PR (eds) (2008) *Bailey & Love's Short Practice of Surgery*, 25th edn, p1252.

3. C ★   OHEM, 4th edn → p536

The patient has acute urinary retention. As he is unable to pass urine, it accumulates in the bladder resulting in discomfort followed by severe pain. The enlarged bladder causes fullness in the suprapubic area and may extend up to umbilicus. It is dull on percussion. The patient requires urgent bladder decompression by urethral catheterization following strict aseptic technique. After releasing the retention, patient may be referred to the on-call urology/surgical team for further management.

A: Abdominal X-ray is not indicated and unhelpful in this situation.

B: IV morphine will not relieve the pain, which requires urinary bladder decompression.

D: This investigation is not indicated.

E: IV fluid will not relieve the condition and may make the pain worse as increased urine formation will distend the urinary bladder even more.

4. D ★   OHEM, 4th edn → p538

The most likely diagnosis is testicular torsion, which is most common between 10 and 25 years of age. The typical presentation is sudden pain in the groin and the lower abdomen.

A: Acute epididymoorchitis typically involves gradual onset of progressive testicular ache with subsequent swelling of the epididymis and testis. There may be a history of dysuria or urethral discharge and pyrexia.

B: Scrotal cellulitis is skin inflammation and presents as local pain and swelling but the testis is normal.

C: In strangulated hernia, the patient usually has an irreducible inguinoscrotal swelling, which may be tender.

E: Ureteric colic may present as unilateral pain with radiation to the loin or towards the testis and is associated with haematuria; scrotal examination is usually normal.

If the diagnosis of testicular torsion is missed, the testis will become necrosed.

Williams NS, Bulstrode CJK, O'Connell PR (eds) (2008) *Bailey & Love's Short Practice of Surgery*, 25th edn, pp1379–80.

5. A ★   OHEM, 4th edn → p543

The most likely diagnosis is a breast abscess. The most likely organism involved is *Staphylococcus aureus,* which causes localized abscess formation. *Staphylococcus epidermidis* (previously *Staphylococcus albus*) causes infection in prostheses or indwelling venous catheters. *Streptococcus faecalis* and *Streptococcus pyogenes* cause wound infections in large bowel surgery. *Streptococcus viridans* is not associated with wound infections.

Breast abscess requires incision and drainage under general anaesthesia.

Williams NS, Bulstrode CJK, O'Connell PR (eds) (2008) *Bailey & Love's Short Practice of Surgery*, 25th edn, pp44–5.

6. A ★   OHEM, 4th edn → p546

The patient most probably has a ruptured AAA. These cases are often missed if not examined properly. The abdomen must be palpated for a tender pulsatile mass. One or both the femoral pulses may be absent. In a healthy elderly person with back pain and signs of systemic compromise, a ruptured AAA must be the first diagnosis to consider. An ultrasound examination in the ED may rapidly help in establishing the diagnosis of AAA. The ultrasound examination is not used to detect rupture, but the diagnosis of an aneurysm may be made and its size may be measured. Spinal X-ray may be arranged if the ultrasound examination is normal and there is suspicion of pathological fracture in the spine.

A KUB X-ray may not be helpful in this situation. Rectal diclofenac is the treatment of ureteric colic. In AAA, a titrated dose of morphine may be given for pain relief. There is no indication for referring this patient to an orthopaedic surgeon.

Williams NS, Bulstrode CJK, O'Connell PR (eds) (2008) *Bailey & Love's Short Practice of Surgery*, 25th edn, p918.

7. D ★ ★ ★   OHEM, 4th edn → p524

The patient has acute pancreatitis, the cause of which is long-standing alcohol misuse. The common biochemistry abnormality is raised serum amylase more than five times of the normal value, raised urea because of dehydration and low calcium level. In addition, the patient may also have a raised WBC, abnormal liver function tests, and hyperglycaemia.

E: The result shows hypercalcaemia with dehydration, which may be possible in acute pancreatitis if hypercalcaemia is a precipitating factor.

8. B ★ ★ ★   OHEM, 4th edn → p545

Patients with chronic venous hypertension associated with varicose veins may have significant haemorrhage from the dilated, thin-walled veins. The haemorrhage may be profuse and cause hypovolaemic shock. Apply a pressure bandage over a non-adherent dressing and elevate the leg to control the haemorrhage. Exclude any arterial disease as this may co-exist. Mostly these measures will stop such bleeding but if it does not the patient will require surgical referral and admission. Applying adrenaline-soaked gauze is not helpful as the bleeding vessels are larger in size than the capillaries, where this treatment is effective. Immediate cauterization in the theatre may be tried if the pressure bandage does not work. There is no role of percutaneous vascular embolization. Injection sclerotherapy is used to treat varicose veins in routine cases in the theatre. It has no role in bleeding varicose veins.

9. E ★ ★ ★ OHEM, 4th edn → pp722–3

The patient probably has an irreducible, painful inguinal hernia, which may be strangulated or obstructed. An abdominal film may be done to check if intestinal obstruction has developed as a result of the obstructed hernia. Such cases should be referred to surgeons for admission and surgery irrespective of the results of the X-ray.

B: This is an surgical emergency. Truss may be given in a small inguinal reducible hernia, not in an emergency such as this.

C and D: Such patients should not be discharged even if the pain or the swelling is reduced or the abdominal film appears to have no sign of intestinal obstruction.

10. D ★ ★ ★ OHEM, 4th edn → p532

The most likely diagnosis is sigmoid volvulus. The plain abdominal film in Fig. 10.2 shows a dilated loop of bowel extending from the left side of the pelvis towards the upper abdomen and sometimes to the right. In caecal volvulus there is a gas-filled ileum and occasionally a distended caecum. Gall stone ileus would cause a paralytic ileus with generalized small intestinal distension. A left obstructed inguinal hernia may cause generalized distension of the gut. Small intestinal volvulus is uncommon and will show features of intestinal obstruction on a plain film of the abdomen.

Williams NS, Bulstrode CJK, O'Connell PR (eds) (2008) *Bailey & Love's Short Practice of Surgery*, 25th edn, pp1195–6.

11. D ★ ★ ★ OHEM, 4th edn → p537

While inserting a catheter, slight resistance may be felt while passing it through the prostatic urethra. Adjusting the angle of the penis by pulling it in a horizontal position between the patient's legs usually sorts the problem. If still unsuccessful, call the senior medical ED staff for help.

A: Application of excessive force may cause trauma to the delicate urethral epithelium, which may result in bleeding from the urethra.

B: Suprapubic catheterization is done by a senior ED staff (consultant level) or preferably by the on-call urology/surgical specialty doctor if urethral catheterization fails.

Surgery

C: Refer to urology in cases when there is significant problem of urine retention and difficult catheterization in spite of repositioning as described above.

E: Catheter introducers are used by urologists. Their use is not recommended in the ED as there is a risk of significant damage to the urethra if they are not inserted properly.

12. E ★ ★ ★   OHEM, 4th edn → p526

The most probable diagnosis is biliary colic. As the pain has settled and patient is not unwell and has normal blood tests, she may be discharged with advice about follow-up and reassessment by her GP, who could arrange ultrasonography or refer for a surgical outpatient appointment. There is no indication for hospital admission and the patient does not require urgent investigation for the same reasons. There is no indication to start antibiotics. The stone in the gallbladder causing biliary colic may cause infection (acute cholecystitis, empyema) or jaundice, if it migrates from the gallbladder to common bile duct, resulting in its obstruction.

Williams NS, Bulstrode CJK, O'Connell PR (eds) (2008) *Bailey & Love's Short Practice of Surgery*, 25th edn, p1120.

Extended Matching Answers

1. A ★   OHEM, 4th edn → p523

This is a real-life scenario in which a ruptured appendix was missed. The patient came back the next day and had surgery. In patients with central abdominal pain, localized tenderness and features of peritonism, appendicitis is still the first diagnosis. There is no other diagnosis in the list of options that could explain all these features.

2. E ★   OHEM, 4th edn → p524

This is a classic history of acute pancreatitis. The main differential is peptic perforation, where the abdominal tenderness will be generalized or some tenderness is expected in the right lower quadrant. However, an erect chest X-ray would be required to exclude peptic perforation. The previous history of gallstones suggests the most likely diagnosis is acute pancreatitis. This is a relatively common but serious cause of abdominal pain in middle-aged and elderly people.

3. H ★   OHEM, 4th edn → p527

The most likely diagnosis in this patient is peptic perforation. Sudden onset of pain with generalized tenderness and rebound + absence of bowel sounds, on the background of NSAIDs possibly points towards peptic perforation. The second possible diagnosis is acute pancreatitis.

4. G ★   OHEM, 4th edn → p530

The most likely diagnosis in this case is mesenteric ischaemia or infarction. Acute mesenteric infarction usually occurs in those >50. It is often heralded by severe, sudden onset of diffuse abdominal pain. Typically, initially the severity of the pain far exceeds the associated physical signs. The pain may radiate to the back. Initially there may be little more than diffuse mild abdominal tenderness. Search for evidence of an embolic source (AF, recent myocardial infarction with high risk of mural thrombus, aortic valve disease, etc.).

5. C ★   OHEM, 4th edn → p532

This man has acute diverticulitis. The prevalence of diverticulitis in the Western world is 60% over the age of 60 years. The condition is found in the sigmoid colon in 90% of cases, but the caecum can also be involved and, on occasion, the entire large bowel can be affected. Diverticulitis is the result of infection of one or more diverticula, usually associated with some pericolitis.

Williams NS, Bulstrode CJK, O'Connell PR (eds) (2008) *Bailey & Love's Short Practice of Surgery*, 25th edn.

Surgery

CHAPTER 11

OPHTHALMOLOGY

'The eye sees only what the mind is prepared to comprehend.'
Henri Bergson

Approximately 2% of ED attendances comprise patients with eye complaints. Most of the time this group of patients is seen by a junior doctor with very little training in thorough and relevant history taking and examination. The majority of such eye problems can be treated in the ED without requiring any intervention from an ophthalmologist. But a few may require immediate action and subsequent referral to the on-call ophthalmologist. Most of the emergencies require a standard approach to history taking followed by an examination, although some (acid or alkali burns) may need immediate treatment, which is given while the assessment is being done.

In ophthalmology, the history will help indicate the part of the eyes to focus on during the physical examination. The following points should be covered in the history:

- Associated trauma
- Pain versus irritation
- Photophobia
- Discharge—colour, quantity and consistency
- Loss of vision
- Pattern and speed of onset of symptoms
- Any past eye problems in the same or the other eye.

During the physical examination always measure VA separately for each eye by using Snellen's chart and document your findings. If the patient wears glasses, these should be kept on during the test. The examination should also include a good look at the eyelids (both from outside and inside), conjunctivae, cornea, pupils and their size and reaction, visual fields, eye movements, and ophthalmoscopy. Do not forget to evert the upper eyelid with the help of a cotton bud as tiny foreign bodies often hide underneath it and their removal will immediate relieve the symptoms—the patient will be very grateful!

Patients with potentially serious pathology requiring *immediate* ophthalmology referral include those with:

- Sudden loss of vision
- New reduction in VA
- Acute red and painful eye (suspect acute glaucoma)
- Penetrating eye injuries
- Chemical burns to the eye
- Suspected iritis, herpes zoster infection, and orbital cellulitis (referral on the same day).

The questions in this chapter cover the common eye emergencies and a few uncommon but serious pathologies. ∎

OPHTHALMOLOGY
SINGLE BEST ANSWERS

1. A 23-year-old man has splashed his left eye with cleansing liquid while cleaning a toilet. The eye is painful and red, and he is finding it difficult to open it. His VA is 6/6 and 6/12 in the right and left eye, respectively. Which is the *single* most appropriate immediate management? ★

A Instilling antibiotic drops immediately

B Instilling the antidote into the eye

C Instilling steroid drops immediately

D Irrigating the eye with saline solution

E Referral to ophthalmologist immediately

2. A 72-year-old man has had a foreign body sensation in both his eyes for the past few days. The eyes are slightly painful and red. The man has had type 1 diabetes for many years. His VA in both eyes is 6/6. The conjunctivae are red and there is yellow coloured, thick discharge present. The corneas and pupils appear normal. Which is the *single* most likely causative organism? ★

A *Chlamydia trachomatis*

B *Klebsiella pneumoniae*

C *Pseudomonas* spp.

D *Staphylococcus aureus*

E *Streptococcus pneumoniae*

3. A 48-year-old healthy woman has noticed redness in her right eye as shown in Fig. 11.1. There is no pain, discharge or photophobia. Her vision is 6/6 in both eyes.

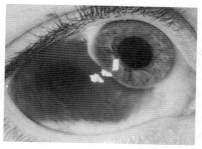

Which is the *single* most appropriate management? ★

A Giving antibiotic ointment

B Giving cycloplegic drops

C Giving steroid drops

D Reassuring the patient and discharging her

E Referral to an ophthalmologist urgently

4. A 32-year-old man has had swelling and redness around his left eye for 3 days (Fig. 11.2). It is now very painful to move the eye. His pulse is 100bpm, BP 145/92mmHg, and temperature 38.2°C.

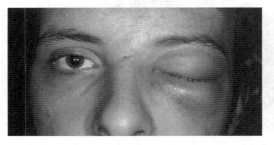

Which is the *single* most appropriate initial management? ★

A Antibiotics – IV

B Antibiotics – oral

C Antibiotics – topical

D CT scan of the orbits

E X-ray of the orbit

5. A 72-year-old man suddenly started having flashing lights in his right eye yesterday. He has been taking ramipril, atenolol, gliclazide, and aspirin for many years. His VA in the right eye is 6/36, the left eye 6/12. The conjunctivae, corneas, and pupils appear normal. The fundus is shown in Fig. 11.3.

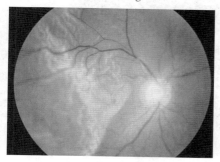

Which is the *single* most likely diagnosis? ★ ★

A Central retinal artery occlusion

B Central retinal vein occlusion

C Retinal detachment

D Vitreous detachment

E Vitreous haemorrhage

6. A 52-year-old man has been having floaters in his right eye for the past few days and today he is unable to see clearly. He has had type 1 diabetes for many years. His VA in the right eye is 6/60, and in the left eye 6/12. The conjunctivae, corneas, and pupils of both eyes appear normal. There is no red reflex. Which is the *single* most appropriate immediate management? ★ ★

A Giving antibiotic ointment

B Giving sodium cromoglicate drops

C Reassurance and discharge

D Repeating the check-up by an ophthalmologist in outpatients

E Urgent referral to ophthalmologist

7. A 38-year-old man brushed his right eye against the corner of a paper while working in his office. His right eye is painful and it hurts more when looking at light. The VA in both eyes is 6/6. After fluorescein staining the cornea appears as shown in Fig. 11.4.

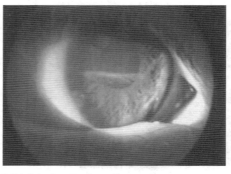

Which is the *single* most appropriate treatment on discharge? ★ ★ ★ ★

A Antibiotic ointment

B Local anaesthetic ointment

C Miotic drops

D No treatment required

E Steroid drops

8. A 28-year-old man has a foreign particle in his left eye, which is painful and red. He is finding it difficult to open this eye. After removing the foreign body, a slit lamp examination is carried out; the eye looks as shown in Fig. 11.5.

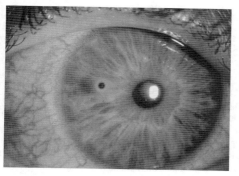

Which is the *single* most appropriate management of the rust stain? ★ ★ ★ ★

A Removal by the ophthalmologist in 72h

B Removal not required, will spontaneously dislodge

C Referral to optician now for removal

D Trying removal in the ED after 1 week

E Trying to remove completely now in the ED

ANSWERS

Single Best Answers

1. D ★   OHEM, 4th edn → p554

Eyes exposed to chemicals are an emergency. The most serious burns can result from contact with an acid or, especially, an alkali. Alkaline solutions penetrate all the layers of the eye causing iritis, anterior and posterior synechia, corneal opacification, cataract, glaucoma, etc. Toilet cleaners usually contain strong acids in various concentrations (e.g. sulfamic acid, hydrochloric acid, phosphoric acid). The eye should be immediately irrigated with lukewarm saline for at least 20min or until the pH of the eye is neutral (7.4) for 30min. Repeated local anaesthesia may be required to enable full irrigation. Washing and local anaesthesia also help in alleviating the pain. There is no antidote available for this scenario. The pH of the eye would need to be measured but immediate management with irrigation will limit the damage of the eye. After cleaning the eye thoroughly examine the eye with slit lamp and refer to an ophthalmologist.

→ www.toxbase.org/Chemicals/Decontamination/Chemicals-Splashed-or-Sprayed-into-the-Eyes/

2. E ★   OHEM, 4th edn → p559

Conjunctivitis may be bacterial, viral, or allergic in aetiology. In acute bacterial conjunctivitis, the bacteria commonly involved are *Streptococcus pneumoniae* and *Haemophilus influenzae*. All the other organisms may cause conjunctivitis but are uncommon. Bacterial infections typically present as red eye, foreign body sensation, eye crusting, and sticky mucopurulent discharge.
Viral infection is the commonest cause of conjunctivitis, presents with redness (more than with the bacterial infection), irritation, and clear discharge. It may start in one eye and spread to the other. It is highly contagious for about 2 weeks after the onset.
Allergic conjunctivitis is usually bilateral, starts with severe itching, redness, and swelling of the eyelids, and may be seasonal or associated with rhinitis.

3. D ★   OHEM, 4th edn → p559

The most probable diagnosis is a subconjunctival haemorrhage, which occurs as a result of rupture of small subconjunctival blood vessels following coughing, vomiting, straining, or any Valsalva manoeuvre. Recurrent episodes may be investigated for an underlying bleeding disorder. If a subconjunctival haemorrhage follows trauma and the lateral extent of the haemorrhage cannot be visualized, consider head injury and associated fractures (orbital or base of skull). If there is no reason to suspect these, reassure the patient and advise them to apply a cold compress for a couple of days. Also advise the patient that it may take 2–3 weeks for the haemorrhage to resolve completely. The other options are not used in the treatment of such a scenario. Antibiotic, cycloplegic, and steroid eye drops are used in various other eye conditions such as bacterial infection, injury, and inflammation. There is no need to refer to ophthalmologist. Referral is only indicated if the condition was associated with photophobia or reduced VA, as this may suggest serious underlying pathology.

4. A ★   OHEM, 4th edn → p558

These features suggest orbital cellulitis (post-septal), which is an emergency. The other features of post-septal cellulitis are proptosis, restrictions of eye movements, and a toxic patient. In preseptal cellulitis, patient may have redness and swelling of eyelids with low-grade fever, which is more common in young children. Both types of cellulitis may follow a sinusitis or local infection following minor skin abrasion or spread of infection from local impetigo. In orbital cellulitis, the patient requires urgent venous access, blood cultures, IV antibiotics (e.g. co-amoxiclav) and urgent referral to the ophthalmologist. The commonest organisms involved are *Streptococcus/Staphylococcus* spp. The patient will require an emergency CT scan of the orbit and brain. Orbital cellulitis may cause cavernous sinus thrombosis or meningitis if not treated urgently. Local antibiotic ointment or oral antibiotics would be inappropriate.

5. C ★★   OHEM, 4th edn → p557

The fundus shows retinal detachment, in which a patient may report premonitory flashing lights or a 'snow-storm' before developing cloudy vision. Macular involvement causes reduced VA. Refer urgently to an ophthalmologist for detailed ophthalmoscopy and urgent surgery.

A: The central retinal artery, a branch of the ophthalmic artery is an end artery. Patients complaint of sudden loss of vision following sudden occlusion of the artery by an embolus. On funduscopy, the retina appears pale with a swollen optic disc and the macula appears as a cherry-red spot.

B: Central vein occlusion is more common that arterial occlusion and may result in painless visual loss of varying degrees depending on the severity of venous obstruction. On funduscopy, the retina has 'stormy sunset appearance' (hyperaemia with engorged veins and adjacent flame-shaped haemorrhages). Cotton wool spots may also be seen.

D: In people >60 years, the vitreous pulls away from the retina giving rise to symptoms similar to retinal detachment or vitreous haemorrhage.

E: Small bleeds may cause floaters with little visual loss but large bleeds may cause painless loss of vision. On ophthalmoscopic examination a reddish haze may been seen in mild cases, and a black reflex in severe cases. It may also be difficult to visualize the fundus.

6. E ★★   OHEM, 4th edn → p557

The most probable diagnosis is a vitreous haemorrhage in which there is bleeding in the preretinal space or in the vitreous cavity. This occurs in patients with diabetes with new vessel formation. The usual complaint is reduced VA and floaters, which are dark spots or strands moving in the visual field in the direction of the preceding eye movement, caused by vitreous blood. Large bleeds may cause further reduction in VA without pain. Refer urgently to an ophthalmologist for detailed ophthalmoscopy and urgent laser coagulation or cryotherapy.

7. A ★★★★ OHEM, 4th edn → p554

The patient has a mild corneal abrasion, which has been stained by the fluorescein and seen by blue light under the slit lamp examination. The patient should be discharged with a prophylactic antibiotic ointment to avoid infection and oral analgesia appropriate to the patient's pain level. Patients should be given topical anaesthesia during clinical examination but they should not be given this to take home, as it anaesthetizes the eye, which leaves it unprotected. While discharging the patient, an eye pad may be applied for about an hour until the local anaesthetic wears off. Otherwise, a dressing on the eye is unnecessary. Avoid using a patch in patients who use contact lens as they run the risk of developing infective keratitis. Wearing a patch also does not promote healing or reduce pain. A mydriatic or cycloplegic drug may be instilled in the eye if the patient is very uncomfortable or has a large corneal abrasion to dilate the pupils and reduce the spasm of iris.

Mydriatics are contraindicated in narrow-angle glaucoma. Miotics, which constrict the pupils, are never given. Steroid drops are not given, as there is no inflammation.

8. A ★ ★ ★ ★ OHEM, 4th edn → p554

Metal foreign bodies occasionally leave a rust stain after removal. Prophylactic antibiotic ointment should be prescribed (whenever there is a breach in the corneal epithelium) and the patient referred to an ophthalmologist for removal of the stain 2–3 days later. This is because the lubricant effect of the antibiotics ointment softens the stain and makes it easier to remove. The rust ring may not dislodge spontaneously and may leave a permanent defect in the cornea. It is inadvisable to remove the ring in the ED either now or after a week, as they are often embedded and removal with a needle may cause deep corneal abrasion.

Ophthalmology

CHAPTER 12

EAR, NOSE, AND THROAT

'A malignant sore throat is a danger, a malignant throat not
sore is worse'

Anon

A variety of ENT disorders present to the ED on a regular
basis and are seen by the ED junior doctors.
The majority of these are benign, but a few may be
life-threatening conditions that require immediate recognition,
rapid assessment, management, and involvement of the ENT
specialist, for example, severe epistaxis (especially posterior
type), acute epiglottitis, angio-oedema, and Ludwig's angina.
Therefore a basic knowledge and an understanding of the
diagnostic features of the common ENT conditions are vital.

It would be impossible to cover the large extent of ENT
conditions presenting to the ED within a small space, hence this
chapter will focus on a few common ENT emergencies that a
newly starting ED doctor would have to deal with on a regular
basis.

There is a wide variety of ENT symptoms depending on the
region affected. However, it is important to keep in mind the red
flag symptoms that signal urgent help of an ENT specialist is
required. Some examples are: sudden unexplained sensorineural
deafness, facial nerve palsy, CSF leak, difficulty swallowing with
toxic appearance, and drooling saliva.

The ENT physical examination is different from other systems
as its components are largely inaccessible, particularly in the
ED. A good headlight, an auroscope, and correct patient
positioning are all important accessories. Although rod lens and
flexible fibreoptic scopes for nasoendoscopy and laryngoscopy
are routine investigative aids, they are outside the realm of
emergency medicine. Most of the diagnosis and management,
however, of ENT emergencies can be achieved by following
simple rules and using basic equipment. If any patient requires

more than an auroscope or standard nasal speculum for a thorough examination, they should be referred to the ENT specialist.

All sorts of foreign bodies may become lodged in the ears, nose, or throat. Most of them cause discomfort but are not life-threatening. A foreign body in the throat may have the potential to compromise the airway—a fact to be borne in mind. A lot of them can be removed in the ED, particularly in adults, but children sometimes may require attention of the ENT specialist depending on their age and the capacity to cooperate. A battery, being a foreign body, needs urgent removal.

One of the commonest ENT emergencies to be seen and managed by ED doctors is epistaxis. A history of an associated coagulation disorder, or treatment with anticoagulation medication for a medical condition, is supremely important, as haemorrhage in such situations may be severe and mortality higher. Such patients should have their haemodynamic status evaluated and resuscitation (ABC) should be initiated. The bleeding can be frightening, causing the patient stress and anxiety, which raises the BP, but the bleeding can be controlled with treatment. ■

SINGLE BEST ANSWERS

1. A 68-year-old healthy man has been bleeding from his left nostril for the last 3h. Application of local pressure has not helped. His pulse is 70bpm and BP 145/85mmHg. There is minimal oozing from the anteroinferior part of the nasal septum. Which is the *single* most appropriate initial management? ★

A Anterior nasal packing

B Balloon catheter insertion

C Cauterizing the vessel

D Commencing IV fluids

E Continuing pressure

2. A 22-year-old man has had a sore throat for 3 days. He has difficulty swallowing, his temperature is 38.2°C, and his tonsils are red and swollen, with visible pus on the surface. Which is the *single* most likely responsible organism? ★

A *Chlamydia pneumoniae*

B *Corynebacterium diphtheriae*

C *Mycoplasma pneumoniae*

D *Staphylococcus aureus*

E *Streptococcus pyogenes*

3. A 30-year-old woman has avulsed her left lower central incisor following a fall to the ground 1h ago. She has brought the tooth with her, wrapped in ice cubes. Which is the *single* most appropriate initial management? ★

A Ask her to self-refer to her general dental practitioner

B Do nothing as the loss is permanent

C Implant the tooth back in the socket

D Refer to her GP for follow-up

E Refer to maxillofacial outpatients

4. A 52-year-old woman has had pain in her left ear for 4 days, associated with a cold and cough. Now on moving her head for few seconds she feels that the room is spinning. Her temperature is 37.7°C. She has a red tympanic membrane with loss of the light reflex and bilateral horizontal nystagmus, which is worsened by changing head position. Which is the *single* most appropriate initial treatment? ★ ★

A Aciclovir

B Amoxicillin

C Beclometasone nasal spray

D Oral prochlorperazine

E Oral pseudoephedrine

5. A 72-year-old healthy woman has been bleeding from her right nostril for the past couple of hours. Her pulse is 62bpm and BP 145/85mmHg. Which is the *single* most likely artery/plexus involved? ★ ★

A Anterior ethmoidal

B Greater palatine

C Kiesselbach

D Posterior ethmoidal

E Sphenopalatine

6. A 74-year-old man has had facial asymmetry for 2 days (Fig. 12.1). He had pain in his right ear just before this problem. He also has loss of sensation in the anterior part of the tongue and he seems to be hearing unusually loudly.

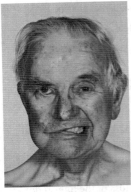

Which is the *single* most likely site of facial nerve involvement? ★ ★

A Cerebellopontine angle

B Cerebral motor cortex

C Parotid gland

D Petrous temporal bone

E Pontine nucleus

7. A 38-year-old man has been having an irritating buzzing sound in the left ear for the past few hours. There is a small, black insect in the external auditory canal. Which is the *single* most appropriate management? ★ ★ ★

A Doing nothing – expect spontaneous expulsion to occur

B Giving antibiotic eardrops four times a day

C Instilling lidocaine before removal of the insect with forceps

D Syringing out with water

E Taking out the insect alive, with forceps

8. A 42-year-old woman has had a persistent sensation of a fishbone stuck in her throat together with pain on swallowing since her dinner last night. The throat looks normal with no visible foreign body on direct visualization with a tongue spatula. Which is the *single* most appropriate immediate management? ★ ★ ★ ★

A Arranging barium swallow

B Arranging a soft tissue lateral neck X-ray

C Discharging the patient after reassurance

D Making an outpatient ENT appointment

E Performing indirect laryngoscopy

9. A 24-year-old man has a swollen, bruised, and bent nose following a punch. The nostrils have some clotted blood and the septum looks normal. Which is the *single* most appropriate management? ★ ★ ★ ★

A Arranging an ENT appointment in 5–7 days

B Arranging for immediate manipulation

C Arranging an X-ray of the nasal bone

D Discharging the patient with reassurance

E Referring to his GP for assessment after 5–7 days if still symptomatic

EAR, NOSE, AND THROAT
ANSWERS

Single Best Answers

1. C ★   OHEM, 4th edn → p568

The most common site of nasal bleeding is from Kiesselbach's plexus in Little's area of the anteroinferior part of the nasal septum. The source of such anterior bleeding must be found and bleeding controlled, such as by silver nitrate cautery under local anaesthesia (by application of a cotton wool pledget or ribbon gauze soaked in 4% topical lidocaine with 1 in 1000 adrenaline (epinephrine) e.g. co-phenylcaine forte). Insertion of a balloon catheter or anterior nasal packing should be reserved for more brisk bleeding or posterior bleeding. Application of pressure will not help. The IV fluids would be required only if the patient is in shock.

For additional information, see the *Oxford Handbook of Clinical Specialties*, 8th edn, p562.

2. E ★   OHEM, 4th edn → p572

The most common cause of bacterial acute tonsillitis is *Streptococcus pyogenes* (group A β-haemolytic streptococcus). Clinically, sore throat is frequently accompanied by fever, headache, and mild dysphagia. The presence of pus on the inflamed tonsils suggests bacterial infection. Other organisms mentioned in the options list may cause infection in the tonsils or pharynx but are uncommon.

For additional information, see the *Oxford Handbook of Clinical Specialties*, 8th edn, p564.

→ http://emedicine.medscape.com/article/228936-overview

3. C ★   OHEM, 4th edn → p578

Avulsed permanent teeth brought to the ED may be suitable for implantation. Milk is the best and most widely available transport medium in which to advise a patient to transport their tooth. The best chance of success lies with early reimplantation (within the first few hours). Handle the tooth as little as possible. Hold it by the crown and clean it gently with 0.9% saline. Orientate the tooth then replace it within the socket using firm pressure. Secure it with a temporary splint. Refer immediately to the on-call dentist/ maxillofacial surgeons for stabilization and prophylactic antibiotics.

4. D ★ ★ OHEM, 4th edn → p565

The most probable diagnosis is vestibular neuronitis following a viral middle ear infection. This follows a febrile illness. Often the patient responds to bed rest, hydration, and symptomatic treatment with prochlorperazine. Improvement occurs in days, though full recovery occurs may require 2–3 weeks. Methylprednisolone may also help but aciclovir or amoxicillin will not. Avoidance of stimulants (caffeine, pseudoephedrine, and nicotine) may ease the symptoms.

For additional information, see the *Oxford Handbook of Clinical Specialties*, 8th edn, p554.

→ http://emedicine.medscape.com/article/856215-overview

5. C ★ ★ OHEM, 4th edn → p568

The most common site of bleeding in anterior epistaxis is Kiesselbach's plexus in Little's area of the anteroinferior part of the nasal septum. The other arteries contribute branches to the plexus. It is important to know the area from where bleeding is occurring while treating such cases as they may often require chemical cauterization.

For additional information, see the *Oxford Handbook of Clinical Specialties*, 8th edn, p562.

6. D ★ ★ OHEM, 4th edn → p574

The facial nerve arises from its nucleus in the pons and leaves the pons to travel past the posterior fossa through the petrous part of the temporal bone to emerge from the stylomastoid foramen and thence traverse the parotid gland, within which it divides into several branches. During its passage through the petrous temporal bone (the facial canal), the facial nerve is accompanied by the chorda tympani (which carries taste sensation from the anterior two-thirds of one half of the tongue) and gives off the nerve to stapedius. Lesions of the temporal part of the facial nerve after the geniculate ganglion therefore produce loss of taste and hyperacusis on the affected side in addition to unilateral facial palsy. Lesions at this level produces a lower motor neurone or infranuclear-type palsy.

A: Lesions of the facial nerve before it enters in to the temporal bone will cause ipsilateral facial weakness with loss of tears, taste, and hyperacusis.

B: Lesions above the facial nerve nucleus causes upper motor neurone or supranuclear-type palsy. Cortical motor fibres to the forehead muscles travel from both motor cortices to each seventh nerve nucleus and therefore, a cortical lesion does not paralyse the forehead muscles. A cortical lesion that produces lower facial weakness is usually associated with a motor deficit of the tongue

295

and weakness of the thumb, fingers, or hand on the ipsilateral side. Taste is not affected in supranuclear lesions.

C: The facial nerve travels between the superficial and deep lobes of the parotid gland in a fibrous plane and divides into two major divisions: temporofacial and cervicofacial, which further divide into five major branches supplying various parts of the face. Therefore, lesions in the nerve at the parotid gland level will affect part of the face depending on the branch that is affected.

E: Lesions at this level are characterized by unilateral sixth nerve palsy, ipsilateral seventh nerve palsy (including the forehead), and contralateral hemiparesis (see Fig. 12.2).

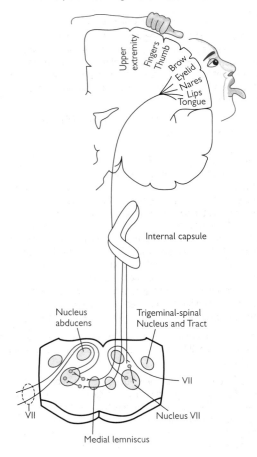

7. C ★★★ OHEM, 4th edn → p562

This is a very uncomfortable situation for the patient and requires immediate removal of the offending insect. First 'drown' the insect in 2% lidocaine to make removal easy. Syringing out an insect may require a few attempts and cause more pain. GA is not required. Holding a live insect with forceps may be cumbersome and it may need to be removed piecemeal. Antibiotic drops are not helpful in expulsion. Microsuction (suction under direct visualization by microsurgery) may be best method to remove the insect, but is usually not available in the ED.

For additional information, see the *Oxford Handbook of Clinical Specialties*, 8th edn, p538.

8. B ★★★★ OHEM, 4th edn → p563

If no foreign body is seen on direct visualization, a soft tissue lateral neck X-ray (to look for prevertebral soft tissue swelling and presence of a fish bone, bearing in mind that not all are radio-opaque) should be requested and then the patient should be referred to ENT for endoscopy. The patient should not be discharged without planned management; making an outpatient referral to ENT will result in unnecessary delays. Endoscopy by an ENT surgeon will be more comfortable for the patient than an indirect laryngoscopy in the ED by a non-specialist. Barium swallow is unhelpful as it may not show any foreign body.

9. A ★★★★ OHEM, 4th edn → p570

The nose is commonly fractured by a direct blow or following a fall onto the face. A nasal fracture is usually accompanied by bleeding for a short period, which often stops by the time the patient is seen in the ED. The diagnosis of a nasal fracture is essentially clinical, based on a history of injury with resultant nasal swelling and tenderness. A normal pink appearing nasal septum excludes the possibility of a septal haematoma, in which case there would be a smooth bulging swelling occluding the nostril. There is no need to arrange an X-ray to corroborate the clinical diagnosis. The X-rays done in the ED are inadequate for this purpose and simply expose the sensitive eyes to radiation. If the nose is deformed or is too swollen, you can arrange for ENT follow-up at 5–7 days so that the nose may be re-examined after settling down of the swelling and if required, manipulation may be performed within 10 days. Referral to a GP may result in a delay for subsequent appropriate corrective intervention. Immediate manipulation is reserved for cases in which there is brisk and persistent bleeding. If a septal haematoma is present, the patient needs to be referred to the on-call ENT specialist.

For additional information, see the *Oxford Handbook of Clinical Specialties*, 8th edn, p560.

Williams NS, Bulstrode CJK, O'Connell PR (eds) (2008) *Bailey & Love's Short Practice of Surgery*, 25th edn. London: Hodder Arnold, p680.

CHAPTER 13

OBSTETRICS AND GYNAECOLOGY

'It is important to know what sort of patient has the disease than what kind of disease the patient has.'

Caleb Parry

O&G is one of the broadest hospital-based specialties, encompassing medicine, surgery, and childbirth; so it is no wonder that O&G patients with a diverse range of symptoms present to the ED on a daily basis. The most common symptoms are PV bleeding, in both pregnant and non-pregnant females, PV discharge, and lower abdominal pain. The majority of these cases are benign and the patient can be discharged after reassurance and arrangement of primary care follow-up, but a few of them may have an underlying life-threatening condition. One classic example is a ruptured ectopic pregnancy. About 10% of females who present to the ED with PV bleeding or abdominal pain in the first trimester of the pregnancy have an ectopic pregnancy. Such patients may present in shock following a catastrophic haemorrhage in the abdomen or arrive at the ED well but collapse in the waiting room. Management of these emergencies requires establishment of IV fluid resuscitation, analgesia, and involvement of an O&G specialist. Such patients are often rushed to the theatre for emergency operation to control the haemorrhage.

In other situations, the normal practice of taking a history and physical examination should be followed. Bear in mind that close attention to privacy and confidentiality is most crucial during the procedure. Interview the patient without the other family members if possible, as the patient may be reluctant to tell the whole story in their presence. Pelvic examination is sometimes painful, undignified, and embarrassing to many patients especially if the examining doctor is a male. This can be avoided to a large extent by explaining the process of examination, and performing it gently in the presence of a chaperone. It must not be forgotten that vaginal bleeding during pregnancy produces maternal distress, for which also the patient will need support.

Patients presenting with lower abdominal pain often have a disease related to the female genital tract or the urinary system. But the lower GI tract may also contribute to the pain and should therefore be included in the differentials. With regard to the reproductive system, there are a few causes of pain during pregnancy. Therefore, the pregnancy test is one of the pivotal investigations in the ED diagnostic process. The presence of pregnancy would signify pregnancy-related problems whereas in its absence the focus would shift to other sources of pain in the reproductive system.

This chapter covers some of the above-mentioned and common situations in the ED and is designed to encourage the reader to broaden their depth of O&G knowledge. ■

OBSTETRICS AND GYNAECOLOGY
SINGLE BEST ANSWERS

1. A 27-year-old woman has been having pain and swelling in her vulva for 2 days (Fig. 13.1). Which is the *single* most appropriate definitive management? ★

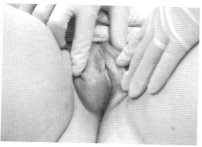

A GP follow-up after analgesia

B Local antibiotic ointment

C Maintenance of personal hygiene

D Oral antibiotics

E Referral to on-call gynaecologist for surgical drainage

2. A 25-year-old woman has had generalized malaise, fever, foul-smelling vaginal discharge and a diffuse erythematous rash for 2 days. Her menstrual period, during which she used tampons, commenced 10 days ago and lasted for 8 days. Her temperature is 38.9°C, pulse rate 110bpm, and BP 100/60mmHg. Which is the *single* most likely organism involved? ★

A *Escherichia coli*

B *Leptospira* spp.

C *Rickettsia rickettsii*

D *Staphylococcus aureus*

E *Streptococcus pyogenes*

3. A 30-year-old woman has attended the ED requesting emergency contraception. She had unprotected sexual intercourse the previous night. Her last menstrual period was 10 days ago. Which is the *single* most appropriate management? ★

A Check the serum β-hCG

B Make an urgent appointment with a local family planning clinic

C Offer insertion of IUCD

D Offer levonorgestrel

E Referral to the on-call gynaecologist

4. A 20-year-old woman has had pelvic pain, purulent vaginal discharge, and nausea for 3 days. She is sexually active. Her temperature is 38.3°C, pulse rate 100bpm, and BP 110/70mmHg. Her abdomen is soft, but her lower abdomen is tender. Cervical motion and adnexal tenderness are identified on bimanual vaginal examination. Which is the *single* most likely causative organism? ★

A Chlamydia trachomatis

B Escherichia coli

C Mycoplasma hominis

D Neisseria gonorrhoeae

E Treponema pallidum

5. A 19-year-old woman has had pain in the lower abdomen, vaginal discharge, and vomiting for 4 days. She is sexually active. Her temperature is 38.3°C, pulse rate 90bpm, and BP 115/70mmHg. The lower abdomen is diffusely tender. Cervical motion and adnexal tenderness are identified on bimanual vaginal examination. Which is the *single* most appropriate initial management? ★

A Arranging urgent pelvic ultrasound scan after taking swabs

B Giving antibiotics after obtaining genital tract swabs and blood for culture

C Giving IV fluids after taking a blood culture

D Referral to a gynaecologist urgently after taking blood count and culture

E Referral to a surgeon after taking blood for count and culture

6. A 64-year-old woman had vaginal bleeding that lasted for 7 days. Her menopause occurred 14 years earlier. Her pulse rate is 70bpm and BP 135/80mmHg. No abdominal or pelvic masses are identified. Pelvic examination reveals a normal cervix and normal-sized uterus with no adnexal pathology. Which is the *single* most appropriate management? ★

A Arranging outpatient CT scan of pelvis

B Giving mefenamic acid and arranging GP follow-up

C High vaginal swab followed by antibiotics

D Reassurance and discharge

E Referral to on-call gynaecologist for further investigation

7. A 24-year-old woman, who is 10 weeks pregnant, has had vaginal bleeding, described as spotting, for 3 days. Her pulse rate is 70bpm and BP 135/80mmHg. The lower abdomen is soft and non-tender. The cervix appears to be closed on speculum examination. Which is the *single* most likely type of miscarriage process? ★

A Complete

B Incomplete

C Inevitable

D Missed

E Threatened

8. A 29-year-old woman, who is 6 weeks pregnant, has been having moderate vaginal bleeding, with clots, for 2 days. Her pulse rate is 70bpm and BP 135/80mmHg. The lower abdomen is soft and non-tender. The cervical os appears closed on speculum examination. Her blood group is O rhesus negative. Which is the *single* most appropriate initial management? ★

A Giving anti-D immunoglobulin

B Reassurance and discharge

C Referral to early pregnancy assessment unit

D Referral to GP for follow-up

E Starting IV fluids

9. A 22-year-old woman has had a sudden onset of severe, left-sided pelvic pain. She also felt faint. Her last menstrual period was 8 weeks ago. Her pulse rate is 110bpm and BP 95/70mmHg. Her left lower abdomen is tender, and her urine pregnancy test is positive. Which is the *single* most appropriate initial management? ★

A Arranging a pelvic ultrasound scan

B Checking the serum β-hCG level

C Giving IV fluids

D Giving morphine orally

E Giving O Rhesus negative blood

10. A 30-year-old, 28 weeks pregnant, woman has been involved in a high-speed road traffic collision. Her pulse rate is 110bpm and BP 100/75mmHg. She has been immobilized on a spinal board. Her left lower abdomen is tender. She has been given oxygen and IV fluids have been started. Which is the *single* most appropriate next management? ★

A Arranging continuous fetal monitoring

B Arranging cross-table trauma series X-rays

C Giving cross-matched blood urgently

D Manually displacing the uterus to the left

E Performing focused abdominal ultrasound scan

Single Best Answers

1. E ★   OHEM, 4th edn → p583

The likely diagnosis is Bartholin's abscess. Secretions from the Bartholin's gland are carried by a duct towards the posterior vagina and lower third of the labia. Obstruction of the duct leads to cystic gland enlargement and sequestration of the gland's secretions. Secondary infection by a variety of lower genital tract organisms leads to abscess formation. Surgical treatment, by incision and drainage under local or general anaesthesia, is recommended and is highly effective. The organisms commonly involved are *Staphylococcus* and *Streptococcus* spp. The other options given are not appropriate.

2. D ★   OHEM, 4th edn → p585

The likely diagnosis is TSS, related to a retained tampon. An exotoxin (called TSS toxin-1) produced by *Staphylococcus aureus* is responsible for more than 80% of tampon-related TSS cases. *Streptococcus pyogenes* (group A streptococcus) is a less frequent cause of tampon-related TSS. Improved health awareness of tampon use and withdrawal of hyperabsorbable tampons have led to a significant reduction in tampon-related TSS cases.

3. D ★   OHEM, 4th edn → p586

There are three options for emergency contraception: levonorgestrel 1.5mg, ulipristal 30mg (a progesterone receptor modulator) or insertion of an IUCD. These options are available in family planning clinics but because the time taken to get to a clinic is unpredictable, it is better to offer levonorgestrel now in order not to miss the appropriate time window.

Hormonal options should be taken as soon as possible after unprotected intercourse to increase efficacy. Levonorgestrel is effective if taken within 72h (3 days) of unprotected intercourse, whereas ulipristal is effective if taken within 120h (5 days) of unprotected intercourse. Levonorgestrel may be dispensed by pharmacists directly to the public as an 'over-the-counter' medication.

Ulipristal is as effective as levonorgestrel, however, both hormonal methods are less effective than insertion of an IUCD. While prescribing hormonal emergency contraception to a patient, it should be explained:

- That the next period may be early or late
- That a barrier method of contraception needs to be used until the next period
- The need to return promptly if any lower abdominal pain occurs because this could signify an ectopic pregnancy.

The IUCD can be inserted up to five days after unprotected intercourse but usually EDs do not have the facility to do so. Prior to IUCD insertion, the patient should be screened for STIs and the insertion should be covered by antibacterial prophylaxis (e.g. azithromycin 1g as a single dose).

→ http://bnf.org/bnf/bnf/current/130057.htm

→ http://bnf.org/bnf/bnf/current/130058.htm

4. A ★   OHEM, 4th edn → p591

The most likely diagnosis is acute pelvic inflammatory disease. An STI ascends from the lower to upper genital tract and causes cervicitis, endometritis, salpingitis, and tubo-ovarian abscess. In the UK, the most common STI is caused by *Chlamydia trachomatis*, and the second commonest is caused by *Neisseria gonorrhoeae*.

→ www.bashh.org/guidelines

5. B ★   OHEM, 4th edn → p591

The most likely diagnosis is acute pelvic inflammatory disease. The commonest organism involved is *Chlamydia trachomatis*. The patient should be given IV antibiotics as soon as possible after obtaining microbiological samples (blood cultures, high vaginal, and cervical swabs). If the expertise to take the swabs correctly from genital tract is not available in the ED, the patient should be referred to the on-call gynaecology team for swabs collection and start antibiotics after taking blood samples. Aggressive IV fluid resuscitation is only necessary if the patient is in shock. A pelvic ultrasound scan could be arranged later to exclude pelvic abscess after initial treatment with antibiotics and referral to on-call gynaecologist.

6. E ★   OHEM, 4th edn → p592

Any patient with postmenopausal PV bleeding despite a normal clinical examination has a high possibility of having adenocarcinoma of the uterus. Thus this patient must be assessed by the on-call gynaecologist. Recommended investigations include pelvic ultrasonography, hysteroscopy, and endometrial biopsy. The patient is not usually admitted, and often referred to a rapid access O&G clinic, as per the national 2-week priority for suspected cancer cases.

7. E ★ OHEM, 4th edn → p602

Miscarriage refers to fetal loss before 24 weeks. Pelvic ultrasonography and clinical examination (particularly whether the cervix is open or closed) help distinguish between the different types of miscarriage. *Threatened miscarriage* refers to vaginal bleeding, viable pregnancy, and closed cervix. If the cervix has dilated, the miscarriage is termed *inevitable*. If the cervix has dilated and products of conception are partially expelled the miscarriage is termed *incomplete*. Total expulsion of products of conception is termed *complete* miscarriage, and the cervix may appear open or closed in this situation. If the fetus dies *in utero* and the cervix is closed, it is termed *missed* miscarriage or *delayed* miscarriage.

8. C ★ OHEM, 4th edn → p602

This is likely to be a threatened miscarriage. The patient may be allowed home, but requires an ultrasound scan (same day or next day) to confirm fetal viability. Many hospitals have an early pregnancy assessment unit, to where such women can be referred. Such units, which are run by O&G doctors, then arrange investigations and follow up the patients as and when necessary. Anti-D is not required for spontaneous or threatened miscarriages below 12 weeks. There is no need for IV fluids as the patient is not in shock. Referral to GP is not appropriate.

9. C ★ OHEM, 4th edn → p604

The most likely diagnosis is a ruptured ectopic pregnancy. Resuscitation needs to be started immediately as the patient is in shock. There is no need to wait for the β-hCG results. An ultrasound scan may be helpful but should not delay the resuscitation, and can be performed after initial resuscitation. Also refer to the on-call gynaecology team as soon as possible as the patient may deteriorate suddenly. There is no need for a group O-negative blood transfusion, as the resuscitation should be initiated with IV fluids, preferably a crystalloid, although blood should be sent for group and save, and antibody testing in case transfusion is urgently required.

→ www.rcog.org.uk/files/rcog-corp/uploaded-files/
GT21ManagementTubalPregnancy2004.pdf

10. D ★ OHEM, 4th edn → p612

Decompressing the inferior vena cava, by manually displacing the uterus to the left, improves venous return and cardiac output by up to 30%. Given there is likely to be a 'C' (i.e. circulation in the ABCD of resuscitation) compromise in this case, this simple intervention should be done immediately. Trauma series X-rays are indicated if cervical, chest, or pelvic injuries are suspected. Remember that the greatest risk from X-rays to the fetus is in early pregnancy. A focused ultrasound scan is helpful to determine free fluid in the abdomen and can check the condition of the fetus. There is no rush to transfuse blood. Initial management is by IV crystalloids. Continuous fetal monitoring may be arranged once the mother has been stabilized by resuscitation through ABCDE.

American College of Surgeons Committee on Trauma (2008) *Advanced Trauma Life Support Manual*, 8th edn. American College of Surgeons.

CHAPTER 14
PSYCHIATRY

'My friend ... care for your psyche ... know thyself, for once we know ourselves, we may learn how to care for ourselves'

Socrates

It is estimated that 1 in 4 people in a year will have some kind of mental health problem, and that mixed anxiety and depression is the most common disorder in the UK. There is an increasing number of mental health patients attending the ED, and a new FY doctor in the ED will encounter such patients from their first shift onwards. The approach to a mental health patient is only marginally different from the approach to those presenting under other specialties. The assessment largely depends on careful history taking and attentively listening to the patient's narrative. There are only a few situations in psychiatry in which a physical examination and investigations are required in the ED to make a diagnosis.

As it would not be possible to cover all the areas of psychiatry which come through the doors of the ED in one chapter, only a few questions have been included here to provide a flavour of the common psychiatric situations that FY1/2s may come across in their early training period. The UK has the highest rate of self-harm in Europe and so one of the most important points is to recognize suicidal patients who can harm themselves seriously and manage them appropriately. If such patients are discharged following an inadequate assessment, they may go on to commit suicide and the attending doctors would have missed the opportunity to support and save them. In this category of patients, when they present to the ED, no matter how minimal is the level of their self-mutilation, it is a serious 'cry' for help. Our job is to listen to the patient and support them with the maximum help we can provide. As it may be difficult to occasionally get to the bottom of the problem, particularly within the time constraints in the ED, a low level of suspicion should be kept to ask for the assistance of the mental health expert.

Self-harm and depression go almost hand in hand. The suicidal rate is higher in depressed patients than in the general population. As 1 in 5 people will become depressed at some time in their lives, recognizing such patients and asking for the mental health expert's help are important to support such patients when they present to the ED. There are situations when the patient with mental health problems has to be treated without their consent and mental health expertise is often necessary to judge the mental capacity of the patient. Along with some of the above issues, this chapter also focuses on the ethical dilemmas that are deeply interrelated with the practice of psychiatry in emergency medicine. ■

SINGLE BEST ANSWERS

1. A 20-year-old woman has attended the ED after taking 10 paracetamol tablets with alcohol. She has been recently separated. Her 4h serum paracetamol level is 10mg/dL. Which is the *single* most appropriate emergency management? ★

A Admitting under the medical team

B Discharging the patient with citalopram

C Giving IV acetylcysteine

D Giving IV thiamine

E Referral for psychiatric opinion

2. A 30-year-old man has attended the ED after drinking 12 pints of lager. His speech is slurred, and he has facial flushing and an unsteady gait. His heart rate is 90bpm, BP 95/75mmHg, respiratory rate 15breaths/min, and bedside capillary glucose 2.1mmol/dL. Which is the *single* most appropriate explanation for his blood glucose level? ★

A Increased glycogenolysis

B Increased glycolysis

C Increased insulin release

D Reduced glucagon release

E Reduced gluconeogenesis

3. A 40-year-old man with long-standing alcohol misuse has attended the ED with restlessness, involuntary shaking of his hands, and sweating. His heart rate is 110bpm, BP 160/100mmHg, respiratory rate 20breaths/min, and temperature 37.9°C. He has been given 10L of oxygen/min. What is the *single* most important feature from the history that will support the diagnosis of delirium tremens? ★

A Believing that he has been drugged by his partner

B Believing that he is the reincarnation of Christ

C Getting a smell of rotten eggs from the oxygen mask

D Panicking after seeing a spider

E Seeing small rats on the walls

4. A 30-year-old man has attended the ED after having 10 pints of lager and a half of bottle of vodka. He opens his eyes on verbal command, makes confused conversation, and localizes pain. His heart rate is 100bpm, BP 130/70mmHg, and respiratory rate 20breaths/min. He has been given 10L of oxygen/min. Which is the *single* most important immediate management? ★

A Arranging endotracheal intubation

B Giving normal saline infusion

C Inserting an oropharyngeal airway

D Performing a bedside glucose test

E Performing a serum ethanol test

5. A 32-year-old man has been brought to the ED by ambulance after being found lying on the street. His heart rate is 100bpm, BP 90/70mmHg, and respiratory rate 12breaths/min. He smells of alcohol. He opens his eyes on application of a painful stimulus, makes incomprehensible sounds, and extends his limbs on stimulation. He has been given 10L of oxygen/min. The bedside glucose test is 4.8mmol/L. Which is the *single* most important immediate management? ★

A Arranging endotracheal intubation

B Giving activated charcoal

C Giving IV 50% dextrose

D Giving IV thiamine

E Giving normal saline infusion

6. A 76-year-old previously healthy man has been agitated for the past few hours. He is accusing the staff in the ED of plotting against him and is trying to climb down from the trolley every now and then. His heart rate is 100bpm, BP 146/90mmHg, respiratory rate 26breaths/min, temperature 37.9°C, and SaO$_2$ on air 92%. Which is the *single* most likely diagnosis? ★

A Alcohol intoxication

B Delirium

C Dementia

D Panic disorder

E Schizophrenia

7. A 73-year-old previously healthy man has had worsening agitation for the past 24h. He is restless and trying to climb down from the trolley. He is able to accurately remember his age, date of birth, the name of the monarch, his home address, the dates of the First World War and identify his wife. Which *single* Abbreviated Mental Test Score does he have? ★

A 4

B 5

C 6

D 7

E 8

8. A 28-year-old woman says she has taken about 140 paracetamol tablets 3h ago. She is refusing to have blood tests or any other treatment, and wishes to go home. What is the *single* most appropriate management? ★

A Calling a senior ED doctor to assess her mental capacity

B Calling the police to detain her under Section 136

C Letting her self-discharge

D Performing blood tests anyway under common law

E Referral to psychiatrist for compulsory hospitalization to treat overdose

9. A 26-year-old woman has been experiencing recurrent agitation, insomnia, and poor concentration. She also has palpitations, shortness of breath, and headaches lasting about 10min. She is worried that she has a serious illness. Her heart rate is 98bpm, BP 126/80mmHg and respiratory rate 30breaths/min. She is breathing heavily. Which is the *single* most appropriate emergency management? ★ ★

A Admitting under on-call medical team

B Giving IV diazepam

C Giving an oral β-blocker

D Listening and explaining followed by reassurance

E Referral to the on-call psychiatrist

10. A 22-year-old woman has attended the ED after making a few cuts to her left forearm with a knife, which followed an argument with her parent. She says she has no intention of harming herself in the future. She has been treated for depression but stopped her medication a few weeks ago. She is separated and now lives alone. Last year she took paracetamol overdose once, which required inpatient hospital treatment. She does not use recreational drugs and is a social alcohol drinker. She has a designated community psychiatric nurse. Which is the *single* most appropriate Modified 'Sad Persons' Scale score? ★ ★ ★

A 4

B 5

C 6

D 7

E 8

ANSWERS

Single Best Answers

1. E ★   OHEM, 4th edn → p630

The patient requires a psychiatric opinion from either the community psychiatric liaison nurse or the on-call psychiatrist.

A: There is no indication for admitting the patient under the medical team as her paracetamol level is below the treatment line.

B: An antidepressant drug should not be started by the ED physician. It should be prescribed by the patient's GP or a psychiatrist if clinically indicated after proper assessment.

C: The serum paracetamol level is below the treatment line, therefore the patient does not require an infusion of acetylcysteine.

D: There is no indication for giving IV thiamine.

2. E ★   OHEM, 4th edn → p643

In the ED, the incidence of alcohol-induced hypoglycaemia is 1–4% and it is more frequently seen in chronic alcoholics. It may present as unconsciousness, convulsions, or other neurological signs. Inhibition of gluconeogenesis, depleted hepatic glycogen stores, reduced plasma cortisol levels, impaired release of growth hormone, and reduced intake of glucose/carbohydrate because of starvation contribute to the mechanism. All other options are therefore obviously incorrect.

Finnel JT, McMicken DB (2010) Alcohol related disease. In: *Rosen's Emergency Medicine: Concepts and Clinical Practice*, 7th edn. Philadelphia: Mosby/Elsevier, p2385.

3. E ★   OHEM, 4th edn → p645

Delirium tremens is a medical emergency associated with significant mortality. This patient has symptoms of alcohol withdrawal. In addition, he may have visual or tactile hallucinations, sinister delusions, disorientation, and confusion. Death may occur from arrhythmia, infection, or cardiovascular collapse. Check bedside glucose, monitor the patient's vital signs, and treat with diazepam if the patient is agitated or having fits. The patient may require treatment in a high-dependency or acute medical unit.

A and B: These are features of disorders of thought processes (psychosis).

C: Olfactory hallucination is a feature of organic brain damage such as tumour, infection, surgery.

D: This is a feature of phobia (zoophobia), the specific phobia about spiders is called arachnophobia.

4. D ★   OHEM, 4th edn → p644

The bedside glucose test must be performed urgently as hypoglycaemia may be a contributory factor in acute alcohol intoxication. If the glucose level is found to be below 4mmol/L, the patient should be given 100mL of 20% or 250mL of 10% dextrose. If he has a history of long-standing alcohol misuse, also give IV thiamine 100mg.

A: The patient has a GCS score of 12/15 (E3+V4+M5); therefore there is no urgency of arranging endotracheal intubation (which is usually done when the GCS score is 8 or below). The patient must have repeated measurement of vital signs and GCS score.

B: The patient may require normal saline infusion to combat dehydration but exclusion of life-threatening hypoglycaemia must receive priority.

C: The patient may not tolerate oropharyngeal insertion as his GCS score is 12/15 and he has preserved oropharyngeal reflexes. It may cause aspiration pneumonia by inducing vomiting.

E: Measurement of ethanol level may be required to know level of toxicity but this not required urgently.

→ www.toxbase.org/Poisons-Index-A-Z/E-Products/
Ethanol--------------/

5. A ★   OHEM, 4th edn → p644

The patient has a GCS score of 7/15 (E2+V2+M3); therefore airway protection and adequate ventilation are required urgently and achieved by performing endotracheal intubation.

C: Activated charcoal cannot be given orally as the patient is obtunded. Even if the patient is able to drink activated charcoal, it is unlikely to be of benefit as ethanol is rapidly absorbed and charcoal does not significantly reduce the rate of its absorption.

C: If the glucose level is found to be below 4 mmol/L, the patient should be given 50 mL of 50% or preferably 250 mL of 10% or

500 mL of 5% dextrose IV as 50% dextrose may cause phlebitis and skin necrosis if extravasated.

D: If the patient has a history of long-standing alcohol misuse, thiamine 100mg IV is indicated, but airway protection is urgent.

E: The patient may require normal saline infusion to combat dehydration but airway protection must receive priority (ABC management).

→ www.toxbase.org/Poisons-Index-A-Z/E-Products/ Ethanol--------------/

6. B ★ OHEM, 4th edn → p136

Delirium is an acute organic reaction characterized by impaired consciousness (overactivity or drowsiness), global disturbance of cognition (memory, orientation, attention, speech, and motor function) and rapid onset with fluctuating course. It is more common among elderly people. Perform a thorough physical examination and administer the Mini-Mental State Examination to establish an underlying cause (sepsis, metabolic, cardiac, neurological, endocrine, etc.).

A: Patients with acute intoxication presents with slurred speech, incoordination, unsteady gait, nystagmus, and facial flushing.

C: Dementia is defined as an acquired progressive decline in intellect, behaviour, and personality. It is irreversible and typically occurs with normal level of consciousness.

D: Functional psychosis is of gradual onset and commonly starts <40 years. Patients have a normal physical examination and vital signs. They are awake and alert, with auditory hallucinations, repetitive activity, rocking and inability to focus.

E: Schizophrenia affects all areas of personal function including thought content and process, perception, speech, mood, motivation, and behaviour. It is characterized by auditory hallucinations, thought withdrawal, insertion or broadcasting, somatic passivity, and delusional perception.

For additional information, see the *Oxford Handbook of Acute Medicine*, 3rd edn, p410, and the *Oxford Handbook Clinical Specialties*, 8th edn, p350.

7. A ★ OHEM, 4th edn → p625

The 10-point Abbreviated Mental Test Score gives a rapid estimate of key cognitive functions, which is helpful in the detection of acute confusional states, dementia, etc. This patient scores 4/10 for age, date of birth, name of the monarch, and dates of the

First World War. The other information is not included in the calculation. See Table 14.1.

Table 14.1 Abbreviated Mental Test Score (Hodkinson, 1972)

Question	Score
What is your age?	1 – for exact age
What is your date of birth?	1 – for date and month correct (not year)
What year is it?	1 – for current year only
What time of day is it?	1 – for nearest hour
What address/place are we in?	1 – for exact address or name of hospital (not just 'in hospital')
Register three-line address and recall at end of test	1 – if correctly registered and recalled
Who is the King or Queen?	1 – for current monarch
What year was World War I?	1 – for either first or last year
Count back from 20 to 1	1 – if no mistakes/corrects self-spontaneously
Identify two people (names/jobs)	1 – if both recognized
Total score/10: <7 is abnormal	

For additional information, see the *Oxford Handbook of Acute Medicine*, 3rd edn, p410.

8. A ★　　　　OHEM, 4th edn → p633

An ED doctor must assess and record the patient's capacity for consent/refusal of treatment (competence). The following factors must be assessed and all must be met to achieve competence:

1. Patient understands information regarding the proposed treatment, is able to retain it, and understands the consequences of refusal of treatment
2. Patient retains that information
3. Patient weighs up the information as part of the process of making a decision
4. Patient communicates the decision.

Record these points separately in the notes. Seek a psychiatric opinion if a mental disorder is suspected to be affecting capacity. If patient attempts to leave (when the patient has capacity), persuade her to stay. If the patient leaves the department, ask the police to bring her back.

B: Section 136 (England) allows a police officer to detain someone found in a public place who appears to be mentally disordered and poses a risk to themselves or members of the public. The police officer's duty is to take the person to a 'place of safety' (usually a designated psychiatric unit, police station, or ED).

C: Persuade her to stay and ask her relatives and nurses to talk to her to accept the treatment.

D: Forcibly taking blood may result in the offence of battery.

E: It is inappropriate to ask the psychiatrist to section such patients for medical treatment. Seek a psychiatric opinion if you suspect an acute mental illness to be affecting the patient's capacity.

In Scotland (**www.sehd.scot.nhs.uk/mels/cel2007_05.pdf**) a registered medical practitioner may grant an emergency detention certificate that authorizes hospital managers to detain someone for 72h.

Fig. 14.1 shows an algorithm for the management of a patient admitted with self-poisoning or deliberate self-harm, who refuses treatment, and is at risk of harm. For a large version of this figure, please visit the book's Online Resource Centre.

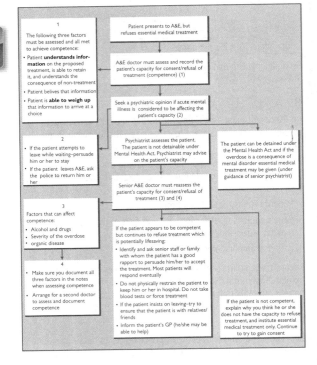

For additional information, see the *Oxford Handbook of Acute Medicine*, 3rd edn, p678.

Mental Health Act 1983.

Mental Health Act 2007.

9. D ★★

The patient is having a panic attack, a period of intense fear, characterized by a constellation of symptoms such as palpitation, trembling or shaking, sense of shortness of breath, tension, agitation, insomnia, sweating, etc. that develop rapidly and reach a peak of intensity in about 10min. The attacks may be spontaneous or situational. Listening may help in reducing the anxiety. Reassure the patient that the headaches are not due to a brain tumour and the palpitations are harmless. Such episodes generally do not last longer than 20–30min. During a period of anxiety, adrenergic responses to stress help survive the situation. But when there are further increases in the anxiety, the adrenergic reaction floods the body system with adrenaline (epinephrine), leading to an exaggerated response that causes the above symptoms. She may also benefit from relaxation training—this involves regulating breathing and muscle tone.

A: The patient does not require inpatient treatment.

B and C: The drugs should not be given by the ED doctors. Sometimes oral diazepam or a β-blocker may be prescribed to help reduce anxiety. If the symptoms are severe and distressing, benzodiazepine (alprazolam or clonazepam) may be given in the ED, which will help in relieving the anxiety and reassuring the patient. Other drugs should be given by a GP or psychiatrist. Beware of the dependence potential of benzodiazepines.

E: There is no indication for referring this patient to the on-call psychiatrist as often the patient settles with explanation. Later the GP may refer her to the community mental health team if symptoms persist.

For additional information, see *the Oxford Handbook of Clinical Specialties*, 8th edn, p344, and the *Oxford Handbook of Psychiatry*, 2nd edn, pp326–31.

10. A ★★★ OHEM, 4th edn → p632

The Modified 'Sad Persons' Scale helps non-psychiatrists to make an assessment of the suicide risk. It may serve as a guide while assessing the need for referral or admission:

- Sex, male: 1
- Age <19 years or >45 years: 1

- Depression or hopelessness: 2
- Previous suicide attempts or psychiatric care: 1
- Excessive alcohol or drug use: 1
- Rational thinking loss (psychotic or organic illness): 2
- Separated, widowed or divorced: 1
- Organized or serious attempt: 2
- No social support: 1
- Stated future intent (determined to repeat or ambivalent): 2

This patient has a score of 4 (depression, previous attempt/psychiatric care and separated).

Interpretation of results:

- <6 may be safe to discharge (depending on circumstances)
- 6–8 probably requires psychiatric consultation
- >8 probably requires hospital admission.

N.B.: It must be remembered that this scale is only a guide and may not be sufficiently reliable in isolation. Other important factors (e.g. using violent methods of self-harming, carrying weapons, patient unable to communicate as a result of overdose or alcohol, etc.) may also require consideration when assessing a patient's suicidal risk.

Hockberger RS, Rothstein RJ (1988) Assessment of suicide potential by nonpsychiatrists using the SAD PERSONS score. *J Emerg Med* **6**(2):99–107.

CHAPTER 15
PAEDIATRIC EMERGENCIES

'Every child should be listened to, no matter how difficult they are to talk to.'

15-year-old girl (quotation taken from findings of research with children undertaken by 11 Million in January 2009 specifically for Lord Laming's report, March 2009: The Protection of Children in England: A Progress Report.)

It is normal in the early days of one's medical career to feel apprehensive on seeing a seriously ill child in the resuscitation room. The effect is compounded by the fact that children of different age groups have different normal clinical parameters and require different drug dosages, volumes of fluids to be transfused, equipment of variable sizes, etc. To deal with the situation safely, various formulae have been developed to calculate the approximate weight of the child, size of the endotracheal tube, etc. The *BNF for Children* should be consulted when there is time to address it; otherwise, use the standard chart of common drug dosages according to the child's body weight, which is freely available in almost every ED in the UK. It should cover most of your concerns when seeing and treating the acutely sick child.

Children compensate well with any underlying serious illness, but there are some subtle symptoms and signs they will usually have in such circumstances. If these are missed, and appropriate management is not given or delayed, a child can suddenly decompensate and go into cardiorespiratory arrest unlike adults, who show gradual deterioration before an arrest. The success rate of return of spontaneous circulation from this situation is poor in children in comparison with adults. Therefore, for clinicians treating children, it is highly rewarding to identify those subtle symptoms and signs and institute the required treatment early on to avoid a catastrophe or a poorer outcome.

There are high-quality videos available at the website www.spottingthesickchild.com for junior doctors on how to diagnose a sick child.

'Be gentle with the young' (Juvenal, Roman poet) is a well-known saying. Yet, for various socioeconomic or personal reasons, children sometimes become victims of adults trying to find an outlet for their anger. The ED is the place where such children are then brought to, with complaints that may raise suspicion of abuse. It is our primary duty to safeguard vulnerable young children and provide them the opportunity and support they require to grow up like every other child. A few questions in this chapter aim to stimulate the thinking of the reader in this area.

The scenarios in this chapter cover a range of diseases a child may present with in the ED, from the highly serious situation of cardiorespiratory arrest to minor limb injuries, including the seriously sick child. The options in the questions and the best response in the answers have been designed to keep the focus on the basics of the management to help the reader grasp the fundamentals. ■

PAEDIATRIC EMERGENCIES
SINGLE BEST ANSWERS

1. A 2-year-old boy has pushed a small button battery into his left nostril. He is physically well and playful. Which is the *single* most appropriate management? ★

A Giving prophylactic antibiotics prior to removal in a week's time

B Leaving it for spontaneous expulsion

C Referral to ENT outpatients in a couple of days for removal

D Referral to an ENT surgeon for immediate removal

E Removal with forceps in the ED

2. A 2-year-old boy has had a fever, cough, and cold for 3 days and is now crying and pulling his left ear. His left tympanic membrane is red and bulging with loss of the light reflex. Which is the *single* most likely organism involved? ★

A *Haemophilus influenzae*

B *Klebsiella pneumoniae*

C *Mycoplasma pneumoniae*

D *Staphylococcus aureus*

E *Streptococcus pyogenes*

3. A 2-year-old boy has been vomiting since yesterday. His mother is worried as he is not feeding but is irritable and very sleepy most of the time. His temperature is 38.8°C, heart rate 160bpm, and capillary refill time 3s; he has purple and red colour spots on the skin which do not disappear on pressure. Which is the *single* most likely organism responsible? ★

A *Escherichia coli*

B Group B β-haemolytic streptococcus (*Streptococcus agalactiae*)

C *Haemophilus influenzae*

D *Listeria monocytogenes*

E *Neisseria meningitidis*

4. A 3-year-old boy has had a fever and has been vomiting since yesterday. He is lethargic and quiet. His temperature is 38.8°C, heart rate 170bpm, capillary refill time 4s, and systolic BP 60mmHg, and he has red to purple coloured rashes all over his body. Three attempts to cannulate him in the foot have failed. Which is the *single* most appropriate way to gain urgent IV access? ★

A Central venous line

B Intraosseous access

C Scalp vein access

D Venous access in the hand

E Venous cut down

5. A 30-year-old woman has just delivered a full-term baby in the ED. The baby has been unresponsive and has had no pulse for the past few minutes. She has received positive pressure ventilation five times after stimulation and suction. CPR has been commenced. Which is the *single* most appropriate chest compression to inflation ratio? ★

A 3:1

B 4:1

C 5:1

D 15:2

E 30:2

6. A 32-year-old woman has just delivered a full-term baby in the ED. The baby has been unresponsive and has had no pulse for the past couple of minutes. She has received positive pressure ventilation five times. CPR has commenced and she requires IV adrenaline (epinephrine). Which is the *single* most appropriate way to obtain venous cannulation? ★

A Elbow

B Femoral

C Hand

D Scalp

E Umbilical

7. A 2-year-old boy has become unresponsive in the ED while waiting to be seen. The nurse has shouted for help. On opening of the airway by head tilt and chin lift, there is no visible foreign body inside the mouth and no sign of breathing. Which is the *single* most appropriate next step? ★

A Arranging tracheal intubation

B Attempting five rescue breaths

C Checking the pulse

D Getting venous access

E Starting chest compressions

8. A 10-month-old boy suddenly developed stridor and severe respiratory distress while eating solid food. He is conscious and unable to cough. The oropharynx is clear on inspection. What is the *single* most appropriate management? ★

A Abdominal thrust

B Back blows

C Chest thrust

D Direct laryngoscopy

E Encouraging coughing

9. A 4-year-old boy suddenly develops severe respiratory distress and stridor, and an erythematous rash all over his body while eating. His mouth and tongue are swollen. He has been given oxygen. What is the *single* most appropriate immediate step to initiate? ★

A Adrenaline (epinephrine) IM

B Chlorphenamine IV

C Hydrocortisone IV

D Normal saline IV

E Salbutamol nebulizer

10. A 6-year-old boy is unresponsive. He has no pulse or breathing effort. The monitor display is shown in Fig. 15.1.

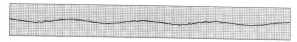

What is the *single* most appropriate immediate management? ★

A Adrenaline (epinephrine)

B Amiodarone

C Atropine

D Magnesium

E Normal saline

11. A 2-year-old boy has had a fever for the last couple of days. He is now irritable, crying, and has vomited a few times. He is reluctant to feed. His pulse rate is 170bpm, respiratory rate 40breaths/min, capillary refill time 5s, oxygen saturation 91%, and temperature 39°C. What is the *single* most appropriate immediate management? ★

A Antibiotics

B Bedside capillary blood glucose

C Blood culture

D Colloids

E Oxygen

12. A 4-year-old boy has been wheezing for the last couple of days. He is breathless and unable to eat or talk. His pulse rate is 150bpm, respiratory rate 50breaths/min, capillary refill time 2s, and oxygen saturation 91%. Which *single* severity of asthma does he have? ★

A Life-threatening

B Mild

C Moderate

D Pre-terminal

E Severe

13. A 3-year-old boy has been wheezing for the last couple of days. He is breathless and unable to eat or talk. His pulse rate is 152bpm, respiratory rate 52breaths/min, capillary refill time 2s, and oxygen saturation 91%. What is the *single* most appropriate immediate management? ★

A β_2-agonist nebulizer

B Intubation

C Magnesium IV

D Normal saline IV

E Steroid IV

14. A 6-month-old girl has had fever, coryza, dry cough, and clear nasal discharge for the past few days. She is now breathless, distressed, and refusing feeds. Her temperature is 38°C, pulse rate 170bpm, respiratory rate 55breaths/min, and oxygen saturation 92%. She has nasal flaring, intercostal recession, and widespread fine crepitations with prolonged expiration. She has been given oxygen and nebulized bronchodilators. The fluorescent antibody binding for respiratory syncytial virus is demonstrated in the nasopharyngeal secretions. What is the *single* most likely outcome? ★

A Asthma

B Bronchiolitis obliterans

C Death

D Full recovery

E Pneumonia

15. A 3-year-old boy has had a fever, cough, and breathlessness for the past few days. His temperature is 39°C, pulse rate 172bpm, respiratory rate 56breaths/min, and oxygen saturation 90%. He looks unwell, is lethargic and his breathing is shallow. He has bilateral air entry with few crackles scattered all over the chest. What is the *single* most appropriate urgent investigation? ★

A Blood culture

B Chest X-ray

C Full blood count

D Sputum culture

E Throat swabs

16. A 2-year-old boy having generalized tonic/clonic seizures for the last couple of minutes has been brought in to the ED. This is the first such episode. His temperature is 39°C. What is the *single* most appropriate immediate investigation? ★

A Bedside capillary blood glucose

B Blood culture

C Capillary blood gas

D Full blood count

E Urine dip

17. A 2-year-old boy having generalized tonic/clonic seizures for the last couple of minutes has been brought in to the ED. He has never had this before and his temperature is 39.2°C. What is the *single* most appropriate immediate management? ★

A Giving IM lorazepam

B Giving IV phenytoin

C Giving rectal diazepam

D Giving rectal paraldehyde

E Inserting an oropharyngeal airway

18. A 2-year-old boy has had generalized tonic/clonic seizures for about a minute or so at home. He is now awake but slightly lethargic in the ED. He has never had a seizure before and has a temperature of 38.3°C. The urine dip test is normal and bedside capillary blood glucose is 5.5mmol/L. What is the *single* most appropriate management? ★

A Admission to children's ward is mandatory

B Can go home with paracetamol and reassurance

C Discharging the patient with oral broad-spectrum antibiotics

D Liaising with GP for future use of diazepam

E Monitoring for a couple of hours in the department before discharge

19. An 8-month-old girl has been irritable and feverish and has been vomiting since yesterday. She is reluctant to feed. After receiving a dose of paracetamol, she is slightly better. A UTI is suspected. What is the *single* most appropriate method of urine collection for investigation? ★

A Attaching a collection bag on the perineum after cleaning with sterile water

B A 'clean-catch' sample into a waiting sterile pot

C Inserting a urinary catheter

D Squeezing the nappy

E Suprapubic aspiration

20. A 5-year-old girl has had pain in the lower abdomen for the last couple of days. She is in discomfort while passing water. The urine dip test report is as follows:

```
Specific gravity 1015; Blood ++; Protein +++;
Sugar -ve; White cells +++; Nitrites ++;
Bilirubin -ve; Ketones +
```

What is the *single* most likely causative organism? ★

A *Escherichia coli*

B *Klebsiella aerogenes*

C *Proteus mirabilis*

D *Pseudomonas aeruginosa*

E *Streptococcus faecalis*

21. A 4-year-old girl has had fever and pain in the lower abdomen for the last couple of days. She was in discomfort while passing water. The urine dip test report in the ED was as follows:

```
Specific gravity 1017; Blood ++; Protein +++;
Sugar -ve; White cells ++; Nitrites ++
```

She was prescribed a 3-day course of oral trimethoprim and discharged. On a follow-up visit 3 days later, the urine culture report has shown growth of *Escherichia coli* sensitive to trimethoprim. The child has responded well to the treatment. What is the *single* most appropriate advice? ★

A Admission to children's ward for further investigation

B Extending the duration of trimethoprim to 7 days

C Follow-up with paediatrics team in the outpatients

D Only investigating further if she has second attack

E Subsequent low-dose antibiotic prophylaxis

22. A 3-year-old girl has had fever and pain in the lower abdomen for the past couple of days. She has been opening her bowel normally and passing water regularly. The urine dip test report in the ED is as follows:

```
Specific gravity 1012; Blood -ve; Protein +;
Sugar -ve; Leucocytes ++; Nitrites -ve;
Bilirubin -ve; Ketones -ve
```

What is the *single* most appropriate management? ★

A Giving antibiotics and send the urine for culture

B Reassuring the parents that there is no urinary infection

C Referral to GP for second urine test after a week

D Referral to paediatrics outpatients for further investigation

E Sending urine for microscopy and culture

23. An 8-month-old girl has had a fever and cold for the past 3 days. She is awake and responds normally. Her temperature is 38.2°C, pulse rate 140bpm, respiratory rate 36breaths/min, capillary refill 2s and oxygen saturation 97%. She has no sign of obvious respiratory distress. What is the *single* most appropriate next step? ★

A Discharging her with 'safety net' advice to parents

B Discharging the patient with oral antibiotics

C Performing a throat swab

D Referral to GP for follow-up

E Referral to paediatricians for inpatient management

24. A 5-year-old girl has pain in her left leg and right thigh after falling from a tree. Both the thigh and leg appear deformed. Her pulse rate is 120bpm, respiratory rate 30breaths/min, and capillary refill 3s. She is receiving 10L oxygen via a non-rebreathing mask. What is the *single* most effective analgesia? ★

A Entonox inhalation

B Femoral nerve block

C Ibuprofen oral

D Morphine IV

E Paracetamol oral

25. A 10-year-old girl has been involved in a road traffic collision when her pushbike was hit by a car. She has multiple injuries and has been given Entonox by the ambulance crew on her way to hospital. What is the *single* most important contraindication to the use of Entonox? ★

A Abdominal injury

B Chest injury

C Limb injury

D Neck injury

E Pelvic injury

26. A 6-year-old boy has had a fall from about 3m (10ft) while climbing a tree. He is opening his eyes on verbal command, his conversation is confused, and he localizes pain. Which *single* GCS best represents his score? ★

A 9

B 10

C 11

D 12

E 13

27. A 2-year-old boy has had a fall while playing. He is reluctant to move the right upper limb. The X-ray is shown in Fig. 15.2.

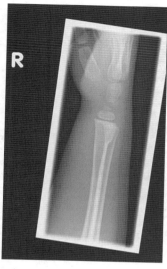

What is the *single* most appropriate management? ★

A Above elbow back slab with follow-up in the next fracture clinic

B Asking the parents to bring back the child in 2 days for a repeat X-ray

C Discharging with advice to go to the GP in a week's time

D Giving a sling and arranging a follow-up in the fracture clinic in 2 weeks time

E Reassuring the parents and discharging with analgesia

28. A 6-month-old boy has been unwell with fever and catarrh for the last few days followed by a rash (Fig. 15.3).

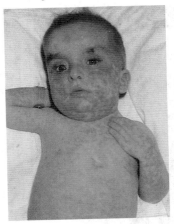

Which is the *single* most likely diagnosis? ★

A Fifth disease

B Kawasaki disease

C Measles

D Roseola infantum

E Rubella

29. A 4-year-old boy has had diarrhoea for 3 days. He is passing liquid stool about four to five times a day. He has had a couple of episodes of vomiting. His sister had a similar episode a couple of weeks ago. He is alert with normal skin colour and texture. His heart rate is 110bpm, respiratory rate 30breaths/min and capillary refill 2s. The extremities are warm. Which is the *single* most appropriate management? ★

A Giving antidiarrhoeal agent

B Initiating IV crystalloid

C Initiating oral rehydration therapy

D Sending blood sample for urea and electrolytes

E Sending stool sample for culture

30. A 6-month-old girl has been brought to the ED by her mother who says that her daughter rolled off the sofa and stopped using the right leg. She has a spiral fracture of the right tibia. Which is the *single* most appropriate immediate management? ★

A Above-knee back slab and fracture clinic appointment

B Admit under orthopaedic surgeons

C Below-knee back slab and fracture clinic appointment

D Discharge with below-knee back slab, analgesia, and GP follow-up

E Referral to on call paediatric registrar after above knee back slab

31. A 4-year-old girl has been brought in to the ED by her stepfather who says she fell astride the handle of her bike (see Fig. 15.4). The pelvic X-ray is normal.

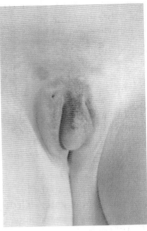

Which is the *single* most appropriate immediate management? ★

A Arranging abdominal and pelvic CT scan

B Discharging the patient with analgesia and GP follow-up

C Giving analgesia and referring to paediatric registrar

D Giving analgesia and referring to surgical registrar

E Reassuring the father and discharging the child

32. A 15-month-old boy has been brought to the ED. According to his 19-year-old mother and her boyfriend, he caught his right arm in his pram and has stopped using it for 3 days. The mother says she thought it would get better on its own. He has a spiral fracture of the right humerus. Which is the *single* most important feature in the history that will suggest a non-accidental injury? ★

A Age of the child

B Age of the mother

C Consistent history of the injury from both the parents

D Mechanism of injury

E Satisfactory explanation of delay in seeking medical help

33. A 14-year-old girl has a compound fracture of the left femur with significant blood loss after falling from a tree. Her heart rate is 130bpm and BP 80/60mmHg. She has been refusing an IV cannula insertion despite her biological mother's consent. Her non-biological father is on his way to the ED. The mother has parental responsibility. What is the *single* most appropriate management? ★

A Applying for a court order

B Following mother's consent

C Inserting the cannula under common law

D Respecting the patient's view

E Waiting for the father's consent

34. An 18-month-old girl has been brought to the ED by her mother with burns on both buttocks. The child was injured 5 days ago when the mother was at work and the child was in the care of the mother's boyfriend. The reason given for the delayed presentation was that she did not have transport. There are multiple bruises of different ages on the back and limbs of the child and what look like cigarette burns. The mother has been informed that the child will be admitted to the children's ward for further investigation. The mother is not happy with the decision. As the nurse turns her back, the mother leaves the department with the child. Which is the *single* most appropriate immediate management? ★ ★ ★ ★

A Doing nothing

B Informing the community child protection nurse

C Informing the GP for follow-up

D Informing the police

E Informing the social services

35. A 12-year-old boy has been brought to the ED after drinking 3 pints of lager with his parents while dining out. After vomiting four times, he is now feeling slightly better. Which is the *single* most appropriate immediate management? ★ ★ ★ ★

A Admitting him under the paediatricians for further investigation

B Discharging him with his parents after advising on alcohol intake

C Discharging the patient after arranging follow up with CAMHS

D Informing the social services

E Referral to GP for follow-up if required

36. A 12-year-old girl has had abdominal pain and vomiting for a couple of days. Her temperature is 37.4°C, heart rate is 170bpm, respiratory rate 55breaths/min with no signs of distress, oxygen saturation (SaO$_2$) 97% on air and capillary refill time 5s. She looks unwell and responds to voice. Her abdomen is soft with minimal generalized tenderness. She has been given a fluid bolus. Which is the *single* most important initial investigation? ★

A Abdominal ultrasound scan

B Bedside capillary blood glucose

C Blood culture

D Chest X-ray

E White cell count

37. A 12-year-old boy has had pain in the front of his right knee for the past week. It is aggravated after playing at school. There is no history of trauma. There is mild tenderness on the tibial tuberosity with pain on extension of the knee against resistance. He has been given suitable analgesia. What is the *single* most appropriate management? ★ ★

A Admitting under the orthopaedics on-call team

B Arranging a full blood count and CRP

C Arranging an orthopaedics outpatient appointment

D Arranging an X-ray of the knee

E Plaster immobilization of the knee

38. A 10-year-old girl has had pain in her right knee for the past few days. Abduction and internal rotation are restricted at the right hip. Her pelvic X-ray is shown in Fig. 15.5.

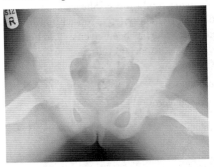

Which is the *single* most appropriate advice? ★ ★ ★ ★

A Admitting under orthopaedics for operation

B Admitting under orthopaedics for skin traction

C Discharging her with reassurance and analgesia

D Giving analgesia and referring to the fracture clinic

E Plaster immobilization and fracture clinic referral

39. A 10-year-old boy has had a twisting injury to his right ankle while playing football. He is reluctant to move and weightbear. His X-ray is shown in Fig. 15.6.

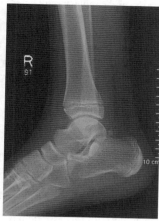

Which *single* Salter–Harris-type injury does he have? ★ ★ ★ ★

A Type I

B Type II

C Type III

D Type IV

E Type V

40. A 2-year-old boy is unresponsive, has no pulse and is not breathing. CPR has been commenced and venous access obtained. His rhythm is asystole. Which is the *single* most appropriate dose of adrenaline (epinephrine; 1:10 000)? ★ ★ ★

A 1.0mL

B 1.2mL

C 1.5mL

D 1.7mL

E 1.9mL

41. An 8-year-old boy has been hit by a car while crossing the road. He has pain in his abdomen and left leg. His pulse rate is 122bpm, respiratory rate 35breaths/min, BP 80/60mmHg, and capillary refill 4s. He has pelvic tenderness and a deformed left leg. He is receiving 10L oxygen via non-rebreathing mask. Which is the *single* most appropriate initial bolus of fluid volume resuscitation? ★ ★ ★ ★

A 200mL

B 240mL

C 280mL

D 300mL

E 320mL

42. A 6-year-old boy has fallen about 3m (10ft) from a climbing frame. He is alert but restless and has pain in his neck, and pins and needles and numbness in the left hand. The cervical spine X-ray is normal. What is the *single* most likely explanation of the sensory symptoms? ★ ★ ★ ★

A Cord injury is common in this age group because of spinal flexibility

B Cord injury is less likely in the presence of normal spine X-rays

C Cord injury may be present in the absence of spine or ligament injury

D Ligamentous injury causing such symptoms is common in this age group

E Such subjective symptoms in young children should be ignored

43. A 2-year-old is reluctant to move her right arm. She was pulled by her brother holding the arm earlier in the day. Which is the *single* most likely explanation for her problem? ★ ★ ★

A Dislocation of the elbow

B Fracture of the olecranon process

C Fracture of the proximal third of the radius

D Subluxation of the radial head

E Supracondylar fracture

44. A 2-year-old girl has been having diarrhoea for 3 days. She has been passing liquid stool about seven to 10 times a day. She has also had a few episodes of vomiting. Her brother had a similar episode a couple of weeks ago. She is responding to voice and has pale skin, and cold hands and feet. Her heart rate is 160bpm, respiratory rate 50breaths/min, and capillary refill 4s. She weighs 12kg. Which is the *single* most appropriate management? ★ ★ ★

A Checking urea and electrolytes before giving treatment

B Giving IV colloid

C Initiating IV crystalloid

D Initiating oral rehydration therapy

E Treating according to the stool microscopy results

45. A 35-year-old woman has just delivered a full-term baby in the ED. The baby has not cried even after 90s following the birth despite providing warmth and stimulation. He has received positive pressure ventilation five times and his heart rate remains at 70bpm. Which is the *single* most appropriate immediate step to be taken? ★ ★ ★ ★

A Give IV adrenaline (epinephrine)

B Giving IV atropine

C Repeating ventilation after applying jaw thrust

D Starting cardiac compression

E Suctioning of the larynx

46. A 6-year-old boy has been wheezing for the last couple of days. He is breathless and unable to eat or talk. His pulse rate is 125bpm, respiratory rate 40breaths/min, oxygen saturation 91%, and PEFR 100L/min. After 30min of the salbutamol nebulizer, he is talking, his heart rate is 135bpm, respiratory rate 42breaths/min, oxygen saturation 92%, and PEFR is 110L/min. He has been given 30mg of prednisolone. What is the *single* most appropriate next management? ★ ★ ★ ★

A Arranging prophylactic endotracheal intubation

B Discharging him with salbutamol inhaler and prednisolone

C Giving IV antibiotics and salbutamol

D Giving a loading dose of IV aminophylline

E Repeating nebulized salbutamol with ipratropium bromide

47. A 2-year-old girl has had a fever and coryza for a few days. She now has a barking cough, hoarseness, and high-pitched inspiratory stridor at rest. She is breathless, distressed, and alert. Her pulse rate is 170bpm, respiratory rate 55breaths/min, and oxygen saturation 91%. She has nasal flaring, intercostal recession and bilateral equal air entry. Which *single* Westley croup score does she have? ★ ★ ★ ★

A 5

B 6

C 7

D 8

E 9

48. An 11-year-old girl has had a twisting injury to her left ankle while running around in the playground. She is reluctant to move the ankle and weightbear. The X-ray is shown in Fig. 15.7.

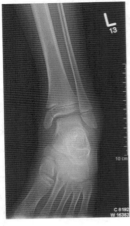

What is the *single* most appropriate management? ★ ★ ★ ★

A Arranging urgent fracture clinic follow-up after applying a back slab

B Discharging him with analgesia, reassurance, and advice

C Follow-up with GP in a week's time after applying Tubigrip

D Referral to outpatient physiotherapy after giving crutches

E Referral to paediatrics for elevation and gradual mobilization as inpatient

49. A 15-year-old has injured his leg while playing football (Fig. 15.8). He is unable weightbear and has pain around his left knee.

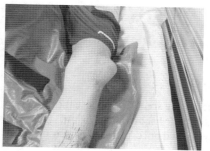

What is the *single* most appropriate management? ★ ★ ★ ★

A Immediate reduction, post reduction X-ray, and immobilization

B Referral to orthopaedics on-call after X-rays

C Tubigrip application, X-ray, and fracture clinic appointment

D X-ray, back slab immobilization, and fracture clinic appointment

E X-ray, reduction, and immobilization

EXTENDED MATCHING QUESTIONS

Diagnosis of rash

For each of the following scenarios, choose the most likely diagnosis from the list of options below.
Each option may be used once, more than once, or not at all.

A Acute lymphoblastic leukaemia

B Acute myeloid leukaemia

C Aplastic anaemia

D Henoch–Schönlein purpura

E Idiopathic thrombocytopenic purpura

F Kawasaki disease

G Measles

H Meningococcal septicaemia

I Physiological purpura

J Rubella

K Trauma

1. A 5-year-old has suddenly developed blue and red spots which remain unchanged on pressure over both thighs and buttocks. He has had a cough and coryza, and pain in knees and ankles for the past week but is otherwise healthy. The spleen or lymph nodes are not palpable. His haemoglobin is 14.5g/dL, platelet count 300×10^9/L, white cell count 11.5×10^9/L, prothrombin time 13s, and APTT 30s.

2. A 4-year-old girl has had a cough and coryza for a week followed by nose bleeds, bilateral conjunctival haemorrhages, and purple coloured spots which do not disappear on pressure. The spleen or lymph nodes are not palpable. The haemoglobin is 14.0g/dL, platelet count 20×10^9/L, white cell count 11.0×10^9/L, prothrombin time 14s, and APTT 32s.

3. A 6-year-old boy attends the ED with red and purple spots which do not disappear on pressure. He has had this for the past couple of days and has been feeling generally unwell for the past few weeks. A couple of courses of antibiotics for a sore throat have not helped. His liver and spleen are palpable. He also has palpable non-tender lymph nodes in the neck. His haemoglobin is 9g/dL, platelet count 48×10^9/L, and white cell count 18×10^9/L.

4. A 5-year-old girl attends the ED following appearance of red and purple spots on the face and conjunctivae which do not disappear on pressure. She has been coughing for the past week and has vomited few times. The lymph nodes are not palpable. Her haemoglobin is 13g/dL, platelet count 200×10^9/L, and white cell count 10×10^9/L. The abdomen is normal on palpation.

5. A 2-year-old girl attends the ED having been unwell for the past few days. She has now developed blue and red spots which do not disappear on pressure; the rash was initially macular and blanching. Both the spleen and lymph nodes are not palpable. Her temperature is 39°C and she is obtunded. Her haemoglobin is 13.5g/dL, platelet count 210×10⁹/L, and white cell count 15×10⁹/L.

Diagnosis of acute abdominal pain in children

For each of the following scenarios, choose the most likely diagnosis from the list of options below.
Each option may be used once, more than once, or not at all.

A Acute appendicitis

B Acute non-specific abdominal pain

C Constipation

D Gastroenteritis

E Infantile hypertrophic pyloric stenosis

F Intestinal obstruction

G Intussusception

 H Meckel's diverticulum

I Right lower lobe pneumonia

J UTI

6. An 8-year-old boy has had pain in the lower abdomen for the past 24h. He is not willing to eat anything and has vomited three times. His temperature is 37.9°C, heart rate 126bpm and respiratory rate 30breaths/min. He has rebound tenderness in the lower abdomen.

7. A 6-year-old boy has had pain in the central abdomen for the past 24h. His bowel opening has been normal. His temperature is 37.2°C, heart rate 110bpm, and respiratory rate 25breaths/min. His abdomen is soft with diffuse, mild tenderness all over. The bowel sounds are normal.

8. A 6-week-old boy has been having projectile vomiting after each feed, which has been gradually getting worse for the past couple of weeks. The vomitus contains milk curd. His temperature is 37.5°C, heart rate 140bpm, and respiratory rate 35breaths/min. There is a non-tender lump palpable in the upper abdomen.

9. A 10-month-old girl has had bouts of severe colicky pain in the abdomen for the past several weeks. In between the episodes she remains well. She has vomited a few times, and the vomitus has contained fluids and bile. Her heart rate is 150bpm, respiratory rate 45breaths/min, and capillary refill 3s. The abdomen is distended and there is a trace of blood on per rectal digital examination.

10. A 15-month-old girl has had colicky pain in the central abdomen for the past 12h. She has opened her bowel about six times since with watery stools and vomited on a couple of occasions. Her heart rate is 130bpm, respiratory rate 30breaths/min, and capillary refill 3s. The abdomen is soft and diffusely tender.

Management of poisoning

For each of the following scenarios, choose the most appropriate immediate step from the list of options below. Each option may be used once, more than once, or not at all.

A Activated charcoal oral

B Allow home

C Endoscopic retrieval

D Gastric lavage

E Induced emesis

F Monitor on the paediatric ward

G Observation in the ED followed by discharge

H Refer to psychiatrist

I Specific antidote

11. A 2-year-old is suspected to have accidentally drunk about 20mL of amoxicillin syrup about 3h ago. She is alert. Her heart rate is 110bpm, respiratory rate 30breaths/min, and capillary refill 2s.

12. A 15-month-old boy has accidentally ingested a mouthful of household bleach an hour ago. He is alert. His heart rate is 120bpm, respiratory rate 35breaths/min, and capillary refill 2s.

13. A 28-month-old boy has accidentally ingested a mouthful of white spirit. His heart rate is 120bpm, respiratory rate 25breaths/min, and capillary refill 2s. The bedside capillary blood glucose is 4.5mmol/L.

14. A 15-year-old girl has taken an unknown number of paracetamol tablets about half an hour ago. She is alert. Her heart rate is 80bpm, respiratory rate 22breaths/min, and capillary refill 2s.

15. A 13-year-old has had half a bottle of vodka during a birthday night out. She opens her eyes to voice, makes confused conversation, and localizes pain. Her heart rate is 80bpm, respiratory rate 20breaths/min, and capillary refill 2s.

ANSWERS

Single Best Answers

1. D ★   OHEM, 4th edn → p215

Button batteries used in small toys are commonly inserted by small children inside their nose. They should be removed by an ENT surgeon as soon as possible because of risk of aspiration if left unobserved. The child may require sedation or general anaesthesia for the procedure.

A: There is no role for prophylactic antibiotics.

B: A battery left inside the nose may cause corrosive burns, bleeding, and sometimes septal perforation within a few weeks so leaving the battery for self-expulsion is not an option.

C: For the reasons mentioned above, urgent removal is required.

E: Attempting removal with forceps in the ED in a 2-year-old boy may cause more trauma inside the nose and distress to the child as well as his parents. It may also push the battery further up in the nose or may be accidentally aspirated, making subsequent removal more difficult.

For additional information, see the *Oxford Handbook of Clinical Specialities*, 8th edn, p560.

→ www.toxbase.org/Poisons-Index-A-Z/B-Products/Batteries/

2. A ★   OHEM, 4th edn → p566

The most common causative pathogens are *Haemophilus influenzae*, *Streptococcus pneumoniae* and *Moraxella (Branhamella) catarrhalis*. *Streptococcus pyogenes*, *Staphylococcus aureus*, *Mycoplasma pneumoniae* and Gram-negative bacteria are much less common.

Some experts believe that the inflammation is caused by viruses in most cases and, therefore, antibiotics are not necessary. The most common virus involved is respiratory syncytial virus, but other viruses (influenza, parainfluenza, etc.) may also cause the inflammation.

Use of pneumococcal vaccine has been effective in reducing the incidence of the otitis media and its complications. Adult infection involves similar organisms.

Hoberman A, Paradise JL (2000) Acute otitis media: Diagnosis and management in the year 2000. *Pediatr Ann* **29**:609.

Pfaff JA, Moore GP (2010) Otolaryngology. In: Marx JA, *et al.* (eds) *Rosen's Emergency Medicine: Concepts and Clinical Practice*, 7th edn. Philadelphia: Mosby/Elsevier, p878.

3. E ★

Meningococcal infection is most prevalent in children under the age of 5y and young adults aged 14y–24y. The bacteria normally live harmlessly at the back of the nose and throat and can be found in around 10% of the population at any one time. Approximately 5% of people who have meningococcal meningitis will die. Meningococcal septicaemia occurs when the meningococcal bacteria enter the bloodstream and multiply uncontrollably. Approximately 20% of cases are fatal, rising to over 50% if the patient develops septic shock prior to receiving medical care (www.meningitisuk.org).

A: The majority of cases of *Escherichia coli* meningitis are caused by a strain called *E. coli* K1. In the UK, most cases of *E. coli* meningitis occur in newborn babies. It can also occur in those with immune systems weakened by AIDS, cancer, diabetes, and other disorders, plus some immunosuppressant drugs. It can also follow a head injury or brain surgery. Infection in newborns occurs during delivery by bacteria normally present in the birth canal. Premature and low-birthweight babies are at a much higher risk. Approximately 20% of newborns die and a large number who survive sustain permanent brain damage. Before 1983, *E. coli* was the most common kind of neonatal meningitis in the UK but GBS meningitis is now more prevalent. Estimates suggest that *E. coli* accounts for around 20% of neonatal meningitis (www.meningitisuk.org).

B: GBS or group B strep, or neonatal meningitis, is the most common cause of severe infection in newborn babies in the UK. Pregnant women can transmit GBS to their newborn babies at birth. The disease in newborns usually occurs in the first week of life —known as 'early-onset'. Babies can also get a slightly less serious 'late-onset' form, which develops a week to a few months after birth. In the UK, about 340 babies a year develop a GBS infection. Babies who survive can be left with speech, hearing, and vision problems as well as learning disabilities. GBS affects

1 in 1000 babies in the UK (the equivalent of 700 babies per year) and sadly 1in 8 babies infected with GBS will die (www.meningitisuk.org).

C: Hib meningitis is caused by the *Haemophilus influenzae* type b bacteria. This was the main cause of meningitis in young children in the UK, before the introduction of the Hib conjugate vaccine in 1992. Following its introduction, there was a 95% fall in cases in children under 1 year of age (www.dh.gov.uk/en/Aboutus/MinistersandDepartmentLeaders/ChiefMedicalOfficer/Archive/ProgressOnPolicy/ProgressBrowsableDocument/DH_5852375).

D: *Listeria* is a bacterium commonly found in certain foods, soil, stream water, and sewage. It occurs mainly in babies, elderly people, and those with immune deficiency conditions. It can be passed from mother to baby during pregnancy or childbirth. Meningitis mainly occurs in babies who get ill 2–3 days after birth, with the most common complications being pneumonia and respiratory distress. Very few cases now occur in the UK. In the main this is due to improved sanitization and increased awareness about the risk of eating unpasteurized milk products, pâtè and undercooked ready-meals in pregnancy. The disease can be very serious, with a death rate of about 30%.

Meningitis can be caused by a number of viruses and bacteria. There are approximately 3500–4000 reported cases of meningitis per year in the UK (www.dh.gov.uk/en/Aboutus/MinistersandDepartmentLeaders/ChiefMedicalOfficer/Archive/ProgressOnPolicy/ProgressBrowsableDocument/DH_5852375)

Also see:

→ www.meningitis.org/disease-info//types-causes/disease-trends

4. B ★   OHEM, 4th edn → p662

When urgent venous access is required and peripheral access in not achieved within 90s or three attempts, whichever is earlier, consider using the intraosseous route. Fluid and drugs given into the medullary cavity of long bones rapidly reach the central venous circulation. Intraosseous access is easy to obtain and can be performed quickly. Central venous line insertion will take longer. Scalp vein access may be difficult in a 3-year-old child, but it is often used in infants. Venous cut down of the long saphenous vein may be performed, but can be time consuming. Peripheral venous access has already been tried and failed. Fig. 15.9 illustrates gaining tibial intraosseous access.

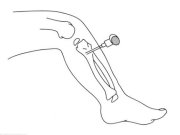

5. A ★   OHEM, 4th edn → p664

In newborns, the chest compression to inflation ratio is 3:1.
The most efficient method of delivering chest compression in
newborns is to grip the chest in both the hands in such a way that
the two thumbs can press on the lower third of the sternum, just
below an imaginary line joining the nipples, with the fingers over the
spine at the back. A ratio of 15:2 is recommended in children above
1 year of age until puberty. The 30:2 ratio is used in adult basic life
support. The other options are not in use.

Appendix 4 shows the Resuscitation Council's newborn basic life
support guidelines.

→ www.resus.org.uk/pages/nls.pdf

6. E ★   OHEM, 4th edn → p667

The easiest and fastest method of obtaining venous access in the
newborn is to cannulate the umbilical vein. Identify the umbilical
vein in the cut umbilical stump: it is the single, large dilated vessel
adjacent to the two constricted arteries. Prepare a 5F gauge catheter
with 0.9% saline and insert it into the umbilical vein for 5 cm.
Suture and secure in place. The other methods are not so rapid when
gain venous access. Fig. 15.10 provides a diagrammatic view of the
cross-section of the umbilicus.

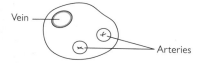

7. B ★   OHEM, 4th edn → p668

The guidelines for paediatrics and adults are different. As the
commonest cause of cardiac arrest in children is hypoxia, the priority
is to treat for hypoxia. In adults, the primary cause of cardiac arrest
in most circumstances is cardiac, therefore the initial treatment
is cardiac compression and defibrillation as soon as possible.
After delivering the five rescue breaths in a child, look for signs of
life. These include any movement, coughing, or normal breathing

(not abnormal gasps or infrequent, irregular breaths). If you check the pulse, take no more than 10 seconds: if the pulse is absent, start cardiac compression at the rate of 100–120/min with a ratio of compression to ventilation of 15:2. Venous access is obtained at a later stage as a part of advanced life support.

Appendix 5 shows the Resuscitation Council's Paediatrics basic life support algorithm, which should be carried out by healthcare professionals. After 1min they should call the resuscitation team and then continue CPR.

→ www.resus.org.uk/pages/pbls.pdf

8. B ★　　　　OHEM, 4th edn → p670

The infant has foreign body obstruction. He is conscious but not able to cough effectively. In such a situation, support the child in a head-down prone position and deliver five sharp back blows with the heel of one hand centrally between the shoulder blades. If this is ineffective, turn the child into the supine position and give five chest thrusts. Abdominal thrusts should not be performed on infants because the liver is still large and there is a potential for serious intra-abdominal organ injury. Direct laryngoscopy should only be performed in an unconscious child with a suspected foreign body obstruction. Appendix 6 shows the Resuscitation Council's paediatric foreign body airway obstruction guidelines 2010.

→ http://www.resus.org.uk/pages/pbls.pdf

9. A ★　　　　OHEM, 4th edn → p672

The boy has developed anaphylaxis following ingestion of food. He has features of potential respiratory tract obstruction (stridor, respiratory distress, swollen mouth and tongue). He should be given 1:1000 adrenaline (epinephrine) 120µg immediately by the IM route. The ∝-agonist effects of adrenaline increase peripheral vascular resistance and reverse peripheral vasodilation, vascular permeability and hypotension. The β-agonist action causes bronchodilation, increases cardiac output and suppresses further mediator release. But beware that excessive ∝- and β-agonist activities may precipitate hypertensive crisis and myocardial ischaemia/infarction, respectively.

B: Chlorphenamine is also used in anaphylaxis at a later stage but in obvious respiratory distress and shock, adrenaline has an immediate action.

C: Hydrocortisone takes a few hours to work and would be given after adrenaline in such a situation to prevent relapse.

D: Normal saline is given if the treatment with adrenaline has not helped and it requires establishment of IV access, which may be difficult in such circumstances and is time consuming. It should be given at a dose of 20mL/kg body weight rapidly.

E: An inhaled β$_2$-agonist such as salbutamol may be used by nebulizer as an adjunctive measure if bronchospasm is severe and does not respond rapidly to other treatment.

Fig. 15.11 shows an anaphylaxis algorithm, published by the Advanced Life Support Group.

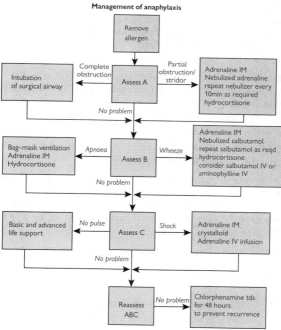

Management of anaphylaxis

Drugs in anaphylaxis	Dosage by age			
	less than 6 months	6 months to 6 years	6–12 years	More than 12 years
Adrenaline IM - pre-hospital practitioners	150µg (0.15mL of 1:1000)		300µg (0.3mL of 1:1000)	500µg (0.5mL of 1:1000)
Adrenaline IM - in-hospital practitioners	10µg/kg 0.1mL/kg of 1:10 000 (infants and young children) or 0.01mL/kg of 1:1000(older children)			
Adrenaline IV	Titrate 1µg/kg			
Crystalloid	20mL/kg			
Chlorphenamine (IM or slow IV)	250µg/kg	2.5mg	5mg	10mg
Hydrocortisone (IM or slow IV)	25mg	50mg	100mg	200mg

* 1µg/kg given 1 minute (range 30 sec to 10min), e.g. 0.5mL/kg of 1:10 000 adrenaline made up to 50mL 0.9% and run at 1mL/min is 1µg/kg/minute

^{1} The strength of IM adrenaline is not intended to be precriptive, 1:1000 or 1:10 000 could be used depending what is practicable. The problem with stricking solely to 1:1000 is that when used in infants and small children, you then drawing up very small volumes.

ALSG: APLS Anophyaxis Algorithm: Updated January 2010

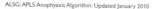

→ www.alsg.org/vle/file.php?file=%2F938%2FAnaphylaxis_
algorithm_120110.pdf

10. A ★   OHEM, 4th edn → p674

The rhythm is asystole. Give basic life support with oxygen followed
by adrenaline (epinephrine) IV/intraosseous 0.1mL/kg 1:10 000
(10µg/kg) body weight every 3–5min. Adrenaline induces
vasoconstriction, increases coronary perfusion pressure, enhances
the contractile state of the heart, stimulates spontaneous
contractions, and increases the intensity of VF so increasing the
likelihood of successful defibrillation.

B: Amiodarone is a membrane-stabilizing antiarrhythmic drug that
increases the duration of the action potential and refractory period in
atrial and ventricular myocardium. An initial IV dose of amiodarone
5mg/kg, diluted in 5% dextrose, should be considered if VF or
pulseless VT persists after the third shock.

C: According to the UK resuscitation guidelines 2010, atropine is no
longer recommended in such situation.

D: Magnesium is a major intracellular cation and serves as a cofactor
in a number of enzymatic reactions. Magnesium treatment is
indicated in children with documented hypomagnesaemia or with
polymorphic VT (*torsade de pointes*), regardless of cause. The dose is
25–50mg/k IV.

E: Normal saline may be given later to treat cardiac arrest due to
suspected hypovolaemia, septic shock, and dehydration.
(See Fig. 15.1.)

11. E ★   OHEM, 4th edn → p688

The child probably has meningitis. He is hypoxic and in shock.
Immediate resuscitation should be commenced. While IV
cannulation is initiated the patient must be given 10L/min
oxygen. After obtaining venous access a blood sample may be taken
for bedside glucose and culture. IV antibiotics (cefotaxime – 80 mg/kg
or ceftriaxone—80 mg/kg body weight) and fluids (20mL/kg body
weight) should follow as soon as venous access been has obtained.

→ www.nice.org.uk/nicemedia/live/13027/49437/49437.pdf

→ www.meningitis.org

12. E ★   OHEM, 4th edn → p700

Features of severe exacerbation are: oxygen saturation <92%, too
breathless to talk or eat, heart rate >125/min (>5 years), >140/min
(2–5 years), respiratory rate >30breaths/min (>5 years), >40breaths/
min (2–5 years), oxygen saturation <92%, peak flow 33–50% and

cannot complete sentence in one breath or too breathless to talk or feed.

A: Features of life-threatening asthma are: oxygen saturation <92%, peak flow <33% of the best predicted value, silent chest, poor respiratory effort, agitation, altered consciousness, confusion, exhaustion, hypotension, and cyanosis.

B: Features of mild asthma are: minimal wheeze, oxygen saturation >92% and absence of respiratory distress.

C: Features of moderate asthma are: oxygen saturation ≥92% and absence of clinical features of severe asthma.

D: This has clinical features of life-threatening asthma with bradycardia.

Clinically it is important to have some idea of severity of asthma so that the treatment could be initiated accordingly.

Table 15.1 details criteria for assessment of severity of acute asthma attacks in children

13. A ★   OHEM, 4th edn → p700

The child has features of severe asthma. He should be given a β$_2$-agonist (salbutamol 2.5mg) immediately driven through oxygen. Continue additional oxygen via face mask or nasal prong.

B: Intubation is not required in this situation, but it is important to call for help, including an intensivist if the condition does not improve or deteriorates.

C: This may be considered in severe cases at a dose of 40mg/kg over 20min IV, but the evidence of benefit is limited.

D: This would require venous access, which may take time. This may be started when the patient is receiving nebuliser.

E. Steroid: the child would also require prednisolone 1–2mg/kg orally or hydrocortisone 4mg/kg IV. Benefit can be apparent within 3–4h.

For additional information, see the *Oxford Handbook of Clinical Specialties*, 8th edn, pp164–5.

→ www.sign.ac.uk/pdf/sign101.pdf (Go to Annex 6)

→ www.brit-thoracic.org.uk/Portals/0/Clinical%20Information/ Asthma/Guidelines/asthma_final2008.pdf

Table 15.1 Criteria for assessment of severity of acute asthma attacks in children

Life-threatening asthma	Any one of the following in a child with severe asthma:	
	Clinical signs	Measurements
	Silent chest Cyanosis Poor respiratory effort Hypotension Exhaustion Confusion	SpO$_2$ <92% PEF <33% best or predicted
Acute severe asthma	Can't complete sentences in one breath or too breathless to talk or feed	
	SpO$_2$ <92%	
	PEF 33–50% best or predicted	
	Pulse >140 in children aged 2–5 years	
	>125 in children aged >5 years	
	Respiration >40 breaths/min aged 2–5 years	
	>30 breaths/min aged 7–5 years	
Moderate asthma exacerbation	Able to talk in sentences	
	SpO$_2$ ≥92%	
	PEF ≥50% best or predicted	
	Heart rate ≤140/min in children aged 2–5 years	
	≤125/min in children >5 years	
	Respiratory rate ≤40/min in children aged 2–5 years	
	≤30/min in children >5 years	

SpO$_2$: oxygen saturation measured by pulse oximetry.
Source: www.sign.ac.uk/pdf/sign101.pdf
www.brit-thoracic.org.uk; www.sign.ac.uk

14. D ★   OHEM, 4th edn → p704

This patient has acute viral bronchiolitis (commonly due to RSV). Most infants recover fully within 2 weeks.

A: Some children may have recurrent episodes of cough and wheeze over the next 3–5 years.

B: Rarely the illness is very severe and results in permanent damage to the airways (bronchiolitis obliterans). This is most likely when infected with adenovirus rather than RSV.

C: This is rare (mortality 1%). Infants with respiratory distress, recurrent apnoeic episodes, persistent acidosis (pH <7.25), and depressed conscious level may require ventilatory support.

E: Pneumonia is uncommon but may occur.

15. B ★ OHEM, 4th edn → p708

The child probably has pneumonia, but other differential diagnoses such as acute bronchiolitis may also be considered. Of patients with acute bronchiolitis, 90% are from the age group 1–9 months; it is rare after infancy.

B: As the classical signs of consolidation (dullness on percussion, decreased breath sounds, and bronchial breathing) are often absent, a chest X-ray is needed. The X-ray may show lobar consolidation, widespread bronchopneumonia or uncommonly cavitations in the lungs. In acute bronchiolitis, the chest X-ray shows hyperinflation of the lungs due to small airway obstruction and air trapping, thus helping in the differential diagnosis. Antibiotics may be started empirically as the pathogen is rarely known at the initial stages.

A: A sample should be sent but the results will only be available a couple of days later to inform further management.

C: This should be performed but is not as helpful as a chest X-ray in initiating the management.

D and E: Same as A.

For additional information, see the *Oxford Handbook of Paediatrics*, p300.

Lissauer T, Clayden G (2001) *Illustrated Textbook of Paediatrics*, 2nd edn. Edinburgh: Mosby.

16. A ★ OHEM, 4th edn → p710

Bedside capillary blood glucose should be done as soon as possible to treat hypoglycaemia if that is causing the fit. Give 10% dextrose IV 5mL/kg body weight (0.5gm/kg).

B: As the child is febrile and having first fit, a blood sample should be sent for culture and sensitivity after the fit has stopped.

C: Capillary blood gas may be required in prolonged fits or status epilepticus where the child required anaesthetic agents to paralyse and ventilate, or is obtunded after having a significant amount of anticonvulsants.

D and E: Full blood count and urine dip are needed once the fit is controlled, for further investigations while finding out the cause of the fit. Urine dip is a particularly essential initial investigation as UTI can be a serious underlying cause of febrile convulsions.

→ www.patient.co.uk/doctor/Febrile-Convulsions.htm

It is important to try to terminate the fit immediately. In the absence of venous access, rectal diazepam is the drug of choice, the dose of which is 0.5mg/kg. Alternately, buccal midazolam may be used in the same dosage (0.5mg/kg).

A: Lorazepam should only be given IV, and it is the drug of choice after obtaining the venous access (dose: 0.1mg/kg).

B: With the child fitting and in the absence of an IV cannula, this is not an option. Moreover, phenytoin is not given as a first line drug to terminate the seizure.

D: Paraldehyde rectally is indicated when the rectal diazepam has not worked and there is no venous access. It should be given as 0.4mL/kg in the same volume of olive oil or 0.9% normal saline.

E: The mouth should not be forced open to insert an oropharyngeal airway if the teeth are clenched during fitting. A nasopharyngeal airway may be tried instead, but may cause bleeding from trauma in young children.

N.B.: A child should also receive paracetamol rectally (20mg/kg) if the temperature is >38°C.

Fig. 15.12 shows an algorithm for management of convulsions, published by the Advanced Life Support Group.

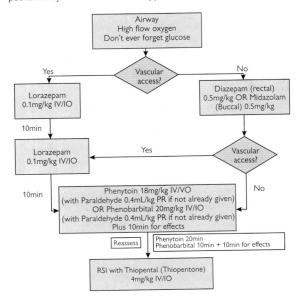

18. A ★   OHEM, 4th edn → p711

All children with a first fit, below the age of 2 years, with serious infections or with an unknown cause of pyrexia should be admitted for septic screening, especially to rule out meningitis.

B: Consider discharging patients who are above 2 years of age with second or subsequent febrile convulsion and obvious benign and treatable cause for pyrexia.

C: Oral antibiotics should be only used if there are specific signs of infection or suspicion of infection (such as a urine infection) with follow-up either with the GP or paediatrics clinic.

D: Liaise with GP to consider arranging for parents to administer rectal diazepam to terminate future febrile fit in the children who are fit for discharge.

E: The first febrile fit patient may be monitored if required before transferring to the ward safely. Children with a previous history of febrile convulsions may be monitored until they are fit to go home with advice as mentioned above.

→ www.patient.co.uk/doctor/Febrile-Convulsions.htm

19. B ★   OHEM, 4th edn → p714

It is essential that urine infections be diagnosed accurately. Contamination of a sample may lead to false-positive results and may subject the child to unnecessary investigations and anxiety to the parents.

A: Cleaning the perineum with sterile water, attaching a collection bag and waiting is the common method used in the ED. (Although may be contaminated with skin flora.)

B: The ideal way to collect the least contaminated urine sample is a 'clean catch'. If this is not successful, then the option B is the next step.

C: Collection using a urinary catheter may be used in seriously ill patients or in whom the previous samples have suggested contamination.

D: Squeezing the wet nappy for a few drops is unreliable as it may be full of contamination.

E: Suprapubic aspiration is reserved for severely ill infants requiring urgent diagnosis.

→ www.nice.org.uk/nicemedia/pdf/CG54fullguideline.pdf

OHEM, 4th edn → p714

UTI is usually the result of bowel flora entering the urinary tract via the urethra. The causative commonest organism is *Escherichia coli*.

B: UTI with *Klebsiella* is uncommon.

C and D: *E. coli* is followed by *Proteus* and *Pseudomonas* in that order.

E: *Streptococcus* spp. is uncommon.

For additional information, see the *Oxford Handbook of Paediatrics*, p366.

21. D ★   OHEM, 4th edn → pp714–5

Children 6 months and older require investigations if they have second or subsequent attacks of lower UTI.

A: Patients do not require inpatient treatment if they are not unwell or have a suspicion of pyelonephritis.

B: The NICE guideline suggests treating with a 3-day course of antibiotics.

C: There is no need of further follow-up in the paediatrics outpatient.

E: Low-dose prophylactic antibiotics are required when patients are waiting for further investigations.

Lissauer T, Clayden G (2001) *Illustrated Textbook of Paediatrics*, 2nd edn. Edinburgh: Mosby.

→ www.nice.org.uk/nicemedia/pdf/CG54fullguideline.pdf

22. E ★

A urine sample should be sent for microscopy and culture. Leucocyte esterase may be indicative of an infection outside the urinary tract, which may need to be managed differently.

A: Antibiotic treatment for a UTI should not be started unless there is good clinical evidence of UTI (for example, obvious urinary symptoms).

B: It is not appropriate to reassure at this stage until a different cause is found or urine microscopy/culture shows a result.

C: The patient should not be referred to a GP. The child should be investigated in the ED or as an inpatient to find the cause of illness.

D: There is no specific indication to attend paediatric outpatients; it may be required if an alternative cause of the abdominal pain is not found or a definite urine infection has been proved.

→ www.nice.org.uk/nicemedia/pdf/CG54fullguideline.pdf (See Tables 4.17, 4.18, and 4.19)

23. A ★   OHEM, 4th edn → p685

The probable diagnosis is a viral coryza. In the traffic light system (Table 15.2) of identifying risk of serious illness, she is in the green part, i.e. low-risk group. Such children can be managed at home. The parents should be advised to keep an eye on the child, watch for signs of dehydration (sunken fontanelle, dry skin and mucus membrane, lack of tears, lack of wet nappies, etc.), give regular fluids, check the child during the night, and give antipyretics.

B: This is a viral illness and antibiotics should not be prescribed.

C: Being a viral disease, throat swab is unhelpful and unnecessary in this scenario.

D: There is no need to refer to GP as it is a self-limiting disease. The parents may attend the GP if the adverse signs mentioned in option A have developed.

E: As above, the child has no signs of serious illness, therefore, may be managed at home with appropriate advice to the parents. Inpatient treatment is not required.

Table 15.2 Traffic light system for identifying risk of serious illness

	Green – low risk	Amber – intermediate risk	Red – high risk
Colour	Normal colour of skin, lips, and tongue	Pallor reported by parent/carer	Pale/mottled/ashen/blue
Activity	• Responds normally to social cues • Content/smiles • Stays awake or awakens quickly • Strong normal cry/not crying	• Not responding normally to social cues • Wakes only with prolonged stimulation • Decreased activity • No smile	• No response to social cues • Appears ill to a healthcare professional • Does not wake or if roused does not stay awake • Weak, high-pitched, or continuous cry
Respiratory		• Nasal flaring • Tachypnoea: RR >50 breaths/minute age 6–12 months RR >40 breaths/minute, age >12 months • Oxygen saturation ≤95% in air • Crackles	• Grunting • Tachypnoea: RR >60 breaths/minute • Moderate or severe chest indrawing

Table 15.2 (Continued)

	Green – low risk	Amber – intermediate risk	Red – high risk
Hydration	• Normal skin and eyes • Moist mucous membranes	• Dry mucous membranes • Poor feeding in infants • CRT ≥3 seconds • Reduced urine output	• Reduced skin turgor
Other	• None of the amber or red symptoms or signs	• Fever for ≥5 days	• Age 0–3 months, temperature ≥38°C • Age 3–6 months, temperature ≥39°C
		• Swelling of a limb or joint • Non-weightbearing/not using an extremity	• Non-blanching rash • Bulging fontanelle • Neck stiffness • Status epilepticus • Focal neurological signs • Focal seizures
		• A new lump >2 cm	• Bile-stained vomiting

Adapted from the NICE guidelines on the feverish child, (CG47, Table 4.1).

24. D ★   OHEM, 4th edn → pp284, 735

IV morphine is the best choice as the dose can be titrated according to the response of the patient.

A: Entonox is a mixture of 50% N_2O and 50% O_2. It is useful to initiate analgesia while splinting a limb or performing minor reductions. The action wears off in a few minutes. It is not suitable for severe, ongoing pain from the fractures.

B: The femoral nerve may be blocked at the femoral triangle by injecting a mixture of lidocaine and bupivacaine for a fracture of the proximal shaft of the femur. If the patient has multiple injuries, morphine is preferred although a femoral nerve block may be added to give local analgesia.

C and E: Oral ibuprofen and paracetamol are given while gaining venous access, but these are inadequate analgesics in such circumstances.

25. B ★   OHEM, 4th edn → p286

Entonox is contraindicated in an undrained pneumothorax because this may turn it into a tension pneumothorax; thus one should be cautious in using the gas in chest injury patients. The other contraindications are: possible pneumocranium following a base of skull fracture, intestinal obstruction, reduced conscious level, and facial injury.

A, C, D, and E: Entonox inhalation is not contraindicated.

26. D ★   OHEM, 4th edn → p739

They 'Eye' and 'Motor' components of the GCS are similar as for adults but a modified 'Verbal score' is used in small children. According to the features above, opening to verbal command is 3, confused/disorientated conversation 4 and localization of pain 5, making it 12. The GCS for children is shown in Table 15.3.

Table 15.3 GCS (children)

	Score
Best eye response	
Eyes open spontaneously	4
Eye opening to verbal command	3
Eye opening to pain	2
No eye opening	1
Best verbal response	
Alert, babbles, coos, words or sentences to usual ability	5
Less than usual ability and/or spontaneous irritable cry	4
Cries inappropriately	3
Occasionally whimpers and/or moans	2
No vocal response	1
Best motor response	
Obeys commands or has normal spontaneous movements	6
Localizes to painful stimuli or withdraws to touch	5
Withdrawal to painful stimuli	4
Abnormal flexion to pain (decorticate)	3
Abnormal extension to pain (decerebrate)	2
No motor response to pain	1
Total	3–15

Paediatric emergencies

There is a buckling in the distal third of the radius, which is a type of incomplete fracture (involving one cortex of the bone) seen in children, and is known as a torus (Latin for a round swelling, or protuberance) or buckle fracture. It is treated by giving analgesia, above elbow back slab, a broad arm sling, and referral for a follow-up in the next fracture clinic referral.

Light TR, Ogden DA, Ogden JA (1984) The anatomy of metaphyseal torus fractures. *Clin Orthop* **188**:103–11.

B: There is no benefit in asking the patient to return to the ED for a repeat X-ray in this case as the diagnosis is obvious. If, despite a strong clinical suspicion, no fracture is seen on X-ray and patient does not improve clinically after analgesia and sling, the child may be asked to return for another X-ray.

C: This is inappropriate advice in this case.

D: This is not an appropriate treatment in children as a recurrent fall may displace the fracture requiring manipulation under general anaesthesia. This significant risk may be avoided by immobilizing the arm in a back slab.

E: This is inappropriate advice. Some form of immobilization for about 3–4 weeks is usually necessary to reduce pain.

The most likely diagnosis is measles. This is a typical history with maculopapular rash, which spreads from behind the ears to downwards on the body. Koplik spots (grain-of-salt like spots) on the buccal mucosa are a pathognomic sign. Measles is caused by a RNA paramyxovirus and has an incubation period of 7–21 days. Since the introduction of an effective vaccine in 1968, the incidence of measles in England and Wales has declined dramatically from 800 000 cases per year in early 1960s to 3000 cases in the 1990s. However, following the recent MMR scare, there has been a surge of measles cases.

A: Fifth disease (Erythrovirus, erythema infectiosum) is usually a mild malar erythema and a rash mainly on the limbs, caused by parvovirus B19.

For additional information, see the *Oxford Handbook of Clinical Specialties*, 8th edn, p142.

B: Kawasaki disease is a multisystem vasculitic disease with fever and exanthema that affects children below 5 years of age; there is a slight male preponderance (male: female = 1.5:1) The cause is unknown. The diagnostic criteria is fever for ≥5 days and at least four of the following criteria: (1) bilateral non-purulent conjunctivitis; (2) neck lymphadenopathy (>1.5cm across); (3) pharyngeal injection, dry fissured lips, strawberry tongue; (4) polymorphous rash especially on trunk; and (5) changes in extremities: arthralgia, palmar erythema or later finger tip desquamation + swelling of hands/feet.

For additional information, see the *Oxford Handbook of Clinical Specialties*, 8th edn, p646.

D: Roseola infantum is caused by human herpesvirus type 6 affecting the age group of 6 months to 2 years; onset is with high fever followed by the discrete erythematous macules, which rarely involve the face and may be associated with lymphadenopathy and irritability.

E: Rubella is caused by a togavirus; the onset is marked by a low-grade fever followed by the appearance of discrete, rose-pink, diffuse, maculopapules, which progress downwards from face and may be associated with tender lymphadenopathy, malaise, and petechiae on the soft palate.

For additional information, see the *Oxford Handbook of Clinical Specialties*, 8th edn, p142, and the *Oxford Handbook of Paediatrics*, p683.

29. C ★   OHEM, 4th edn → p230

Although the child has diarrhoea and vomiting, he is well with a normal heart rate and capillary refill, and is not clinically dehydrated (Table 15.4). Therefore, it is prudent to initiate oral rehydration therapy with available formulations. The usual dose is 200mL after each stool. Frequent sips are better tolerated than large volume of drinks.

A: Antidiarrhoeal agents are not used in children for acute gastroenteritis.

B: There is no indication for giving IV crystalloid or colloid.

D: Do not perform routine blood biochemistry. Measure plasma sodium, potassium, urea, creatinine and glucose concentrations if:

- IV fluid therapy is required or
- There are symptoms and/or signs that suggest hypernatraemia (jittery movements, increased muscle tone, hyperreflexia, convulsions, drowsiness or coma).

Measure venous blood acid–base status and chloride concentration if shock is suspected or confirmed (see the NICE weblink below).

E: The indications for sending stool culture are:

- Suspected septicaemia
- Blood and/or mucus in the stool
- The child is immunocompromised.

Table 15.4 Symptoms and signs of clinical dehydration and shock

| | Increasing severity of dehydration $\longrightarrow$ | | |
	No clinically detectable dehydration	Clinical dehydration	Clinical shock
Symptoms (remote and face-to-face assessments)	Appears well	Appears to be unwell or deteriorating	–
	Alert and responsive	Altered responsiveness (for example, irritable, lethargic)	Decreased level of consciousness
	Normal urine output	Decreased urine output	–
	Skin colour unchanged	Skin colour unchanged	Pale or mottled skin
	Warm extremities	Warm extremities	Cold extremities
Signs (face-to-face assessments)	Alert and responsive	Altered responsiveness (for example, irritable, lethargic)	Decreased level of consciousness
	Skin colour unchanged	Skin colour unchanged	Pale or mottled skin
	Warm extremities	Warm extremities	Cold extremities
	Eyes not sunken	Sunken eyes	–
	Moist mucous membranes (except after a drink)	Dry mucous membranes (except for 'mouth breather')	–
	Normal heart rate	Tachycardia	Tachycardia
	Normal breathing pattern	Tachypnoea	Tachypnoea
	Normal peripheral pulses	Normal peripheral pulses	Weak peripheral pulses
	Normal capillary refill time	Normal capillary refill time	Prolonged capillary refill time
	Normal skin turgor	Reduced skin turgor	–
	Normal blood pressure	Normal blood pressure	Hypotension (decompensated shock)

Source: NICE (2009) *Diarrhoea and vomiting caused by gastroenteritis: diagnosis, assessment and management in children younger than 5 years.* London: NICE.

→ www.nice.org.uk/nicemedia/pdf/CG84FullGuideline.pdf

30. E ★   OHEM, 4th edn → pp752–7

Although tibial fractures may occur in children <3 years of age who fall, the mechanism of injury is not forceful enough to cause a fracture of the tibia. A spiral fracture of the long bone in this case denotes a forceful squeeze of the leg. There should be a suspicion of non-accidental injury and thus referral to the on-call paediatric registrar for admission and further investigation. Social services should also be involved by the on-call paediatric team to investigate the social situation.

A: An above-knee back slab is the treatment in the ED, but she should by followed by the orthopaedics team in the paediatrics ward after admitting the child.

B: This is inappropriate as the child should be admitted under a paediatrician to exclude non-accidental injury. The orthopaedic surgeons should be involved in the management of the fracture.

C and D: These are inappropriate for the reasons mentioned above.

For additional information, see the *Oxford Handbook of Clinical Specialties*, 8th edn, p146.

→ www.nice.org.uk/nicemedia/live/12183/44954/44954.pdf

31. C ★   OHEM, 4th edn → pp752–7

The suspected mechanism of injury is sexual abuse. All children with genital injury should be reviewed by a senior doctor in the ED. Therefore the child should be admitted under paediatric care and with involvement of social services for further investigation.

A: CT scan of the abdomen may be required if intraabdominal injury is suspected.

B and E: These are inappropriate management plans.

D: Surgical advice may be obtained on the paediatric ward if required.

→ www.nice.org.uk/nicemedia/live/12183/44954/44954.pdf

32. D ★   OHEM, 4th edn → p724

It is unusual to have long bone fractures in a child <3 years of age. Spiral fracture in a long bone is indicative of the application of a squeezing force. It is important to ensure that child's development correlates with the mechanism of injury.

The following additional features in the history in general should alert the doctor to the possibility of child abuse:

- Injuries inconsistent with the history given
- Changing history of injury
- Vague history, lacking details
- Delay in seeking medical attention without satisfactory explanation
- Abnormal parental attitude towards the child
- Attitude and behaviour of child (i.e. passive, aggressive, etc.)
- Frequent ED attendances.

Occasionally, children will provide an account of abuse.

During physical examination, the type of injury may provide a clue:

- Bruising in unusual sites (medial aspect of upper arm or thighs)
- Multiple bruising of different ages
- Injury imprints such as finger, belt, stick marks, etc.
- Human bite marks
- Torn frenulum of the upper lip
- Perineal wounds and burns
- Cigarette burns.

A: Children of all age groups may suffer from abuse, which may be physical, sexual, emotional, poisoning, neglect, etc. Age is correlated with other factors in determining the possibility of the non-accidental injury.

B: Age of the mother generally does not provide a clue.

C and E: See above.

→ www.nice.org.uk/nicemedia/live/12183/44954/44954.pdf

Ethical aspects of confidentiality and sharing information is explained in the *Every Child Matters* document (Appendix 3) available at the following website: <WEB>www.dcsf.gov.uk/everychildmatters/resources-and-practice/IG00182/

For fractures in children, see <WEB>www.nspcc.org.uk/Inform/publications/downloads/fracturesinchildren_wdf48020.pdf

33. B ★

Children under the age of 16 if judged 'Fraser competent' (formerly 'Gillick competent') can consent to treatment but cannot withhold treatment. As in general a parent with parental responsibility should consent in such a situation. Parental responsibility is defined as 'all rights, duties, powers, responsibilities, and authority which by law a parent has in relation to the child and his property. Parental responsibility is automatically given to the mother. With regards to father's responsibility see E.

A: A court order is generally sought for long-term treatment. In the emergency it may take time (few hours) to obtain the court order.

C: Under common law, a doctor can provide the minimum appropriate treatment to save life in an emergency situation when the patient is not able to give consent (unconscious).

D: As in B.

E: The mother has parental responsibility. The father has parental responsibility if he:

- And the mother were married at the child's birth
- Is unmarried but his name is registered on birth certificate (after December 2003)
- Is unmarried and entered into a parental responsibility agreement with the mother
- Is unmarried and obtained a court order for parental responsibility
- Is unmarried and obtained a Residence Order
- is unmarried and marries the mother.

For additional information, see the *Oxford Handbook of Paediatrics*, pp104–107, 418, 1008.

→ www.gmc-uk.org/guidance/ethical_guidance/consent_guidance_common_law.asp#Children

34. D ★★★★

There is likelihood of serious harm to the child, so immediate safety of the child must be secured. The police have the power to return the child to hospital for inpatient admission, further investigation, and treatment. The police also have the power to remove a child to a suitable safe place in case of an emergency. This is used only in exceptional circumstances where there is insufficient time to seek an emergency police protection order for the reason relating to the immediate safety of the child. This police protection order lasts for 72h.

A: There is sufficient evidence in the history and physical examination that the child may be subjected to serious harm. Therefore, doing nothing is not an option. The doctor and paediatric senior nurses must act quickly in the ED to recover the child for safety.

B: There is a designated child protection/safeguarding nurse in secondary care who liaises with various organizations and must be informed when such cases present in the ED. The community child protection nurse plays an important role in the community and the safeguarding nurse base in the hospital.

C: The GP may be informed about the incident, particularly if the mother and the child cannot be found at their designated home address. But it is important that the child should be returned to hospital as a place of safety.

E: The social services play a vital role in child protection issues and lead investigation of child abuse as a single agency or with the police as a joint agency investigation. A senior social worker is identified to carry out initial and core assessments in the community. After the child is admitted to hospital, the child protection nurse subsequently involves a social worker in further investigations.

For additional information, see the *Oxford Handbook of Paediatrics*, pp970–84.

→ http://publications.dcsf.gov.uk/default.aspx?PageFunction=productdetails&PageMode=publications&ProductId=DCSF-00304-2010

→ http://publications.everychildmatters.gov.uk/eOrderingDownload/HC-330.pdf

35. A ★★★★

The child still requires observation and possibly intravascular rehydration. It is against the law for children under 18 to consume alcohol in licensed premises with one exception – 16–17 year olds accompanied by an adult can drink but not buy beer, wine, and cider with a table meal. The child also requires admission for investigation with regards to child neglect/abuse. Further investigation of parental capacity is also required.

B: As mentioned above, it is not safe to discharge the child on clinical as well as child protection grounds. If clinically safe, in circumstances when the child has one-off alcohol consumption with friends, the child may be discharged home if the parents demonstrate adequate responsibility.

C: The child cannot be discharged until investigated as mentioned in A. The CAMHS team may be involved on the wards if required.

D: The ED is not required to inform social services at this stage but this may be done later following admission if deemed appropriate.

E: The GP may be informed but follow-up may not be essential by the GP.

For additional information, see the *Oxford Handbook of Paediatrics*, p778.

→ www.direct.gov.uk/en/parents/yourchildshealthandsafety/worriedabout/dg_10026211

36. B ★ OHEM, 4th edn → pp154, 713

The child has DKA. Any unwell child in the ED must have bedside capillary glucose performed along with the assessment of ABCDE. Often the acronym is used as ABCDEFG (Don't Ever Forget Glucose). The incidence of type 1 diabetes mellitus is 10/100 000 children and more common in children <4 years of age. In established type 1 diabetes, the frequency of DKA is about 1–10% per patient per year. Although uncommon, the diagnosis is often mistaken to be respiratory illness, hyperventilation, or acute appendicitis.

DKA is caused by a decrease in effective circulating insulin associated with an increase in counter-regulatory hormones (glucagon, catecholamines, cortisol and growth hormone). This results in raised glucose production by the liver and kidney and impaired peripheral glucose utilization, causing hyperglycaemia and hyperosmolality. Metabolic acidosis and ketonaemia occurs as a consequence of increased lipolysis and ketone body (acetoacetate and β-hydroxybutyrate) production. Hyperglycaemia and acidosis causes osmotic diuresis, dehydration, and obligate loss of electrolytes. Ketoacid accumulation also induces an ileus, resulting in nausea and vomiting, and an exacerbation of the dehydration.

Clinical examination must include assessment of the degree of dehydration, level of consciousness, evidence of cerebral oedema, possible source of infection, and calculation of body weight. The child should be treated by normal saline infusion (20mL/kg) if in shock and insulin infusion. The risk of DKA in established type 1 diabetes mellitus is increased in children with:

- Poor metabolic control
- Past episodes of DKA
- Peripubertal and adolescent girls
- Psychiatric disorders (eating disorders)
- Difficult family circumstances.

The mortality rate for DKA is 0.15–0.31%, and 57–87% of all DKA related deaths are attributable to cerebral oedema.

A: Abdominal ultrasound scan may be done later if an abdominal pathology is suspected, but is not important in this case.

C: The patient is apyrexial, therefore, there is no urgency for sending blood for culture. However, if sepsis is suspected to be the precipitating factor, a sample should be sent but the results will only be available a couple of days later.

D: There is no obvious sign of respiratory tract infection, so this may not be needed urgently. To determine the source of infection a chest X-ray may be requested if sepsis is suspected as a precipitating factor of DKA.

E: White cell count is an important baseline investigation, which should be done. But instant capillary blood glucose is more important to initiate the treatment immediately.

For additional information, see the *Oxford Handbook of Paediatrics*, pp104–107, 418.

37. C ★ ★   OHEM, 4th edn → p730

The boy has traction apophysitis of the tibial attachment of the patellar tendon. This condition is also known as Osgood–Schlatter's disease or osteochondritis of tibial tuberosity and affects children aged 10–15 years with a boys: girls ratio of 3:1. It is a type of overuse syndrome related to excessive physical activity resulting in detachment of a cartilage fragment from the tibial tuberosity. This is typically bilateral in 25–50% of patients. Most cases resolve with a reduction in physical activity, non-steroidal anti-inflammatory analgesics, rest, ice and follow-up in orthopaedics outpatients. Sometimes patients who cannot comply with the above treatment may require plaster immobilization for 6 weeks.

A: There is no indication for admission to hospital.

B: There is no indication for these tests.

D: X-rays are often normal and non-diagnostic. The diagnosis is clinical not radiological. A plain X-ray can be used to exclude other diagnosis (tumours, infections, avulsion fractures, etc.) but generally is not required.

E: Plaster immobilization of the knee is not required at this stage. If the condition fails to resolve after several months of treatment as mentioned in D, immobilization of the knee may be indicated.

→ www.cks.nhs.uk/osgood_schlatters_disease#405510006

38. A ★ ★ ★ ★ *OHEM, 4th edn* → p728

This is a case of slipped upper femoral epiphysis in the right hip, with an incidence of 30–60/100 000 children per year; it is three times more common in the boys in the age group of 10–17 years. The peak age for boys is 13 years and for girls 11.5 years. The pain in the hip or a referred pain in the knee may develop suddenly or gradually. There may be a history of trauma. Standard pelvic AP view X-rays may not show small slips, therefore a frog-leg lateral pelvic views (as in the above film) must be obtained. The patient must be referred to the orthopaedic on-call team for internal fixation ± manipulation.

All the other options are inappropriate.

N.B.: Always examine the hips when a patient presents with knee pain.

39. B ★ ★ ★ ★ OHEM, 4th edn → p740–1

Epiphyseal injuries at the end of the long bones are classified into five types in the Salter–Harris classification (Fig. 15.13).

Type I: The separation or slippage of epiphysis on metaphysis.

Type II: A small piece of metaphysis separates with the epiphysis (as in Fig. 15.7).

Type III: A vertical fracture thorough the epiphysis and epiphyseal plate.

Type IV: A fracture, which extends from the metaphysis through the epiphysis and epiphyseal plate involving the articular surface.

Type V: A crushed injury to the epiphyseal plate.

The risks of long-term growth problems are lower in types I and II undisplaced injuries than types III–V injuries.

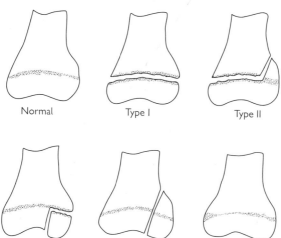

Normal   Type I   Type II

Type III   Type IV   Type V

40. B ★ ★ ★   OHEM, 4th edn → pp666, 674

Between 1 and 10 years of age, the approximate body weight is calculated by the following formula:

Weight in kg = (age in years + 4) × 2.

In this case the probable weight of the child is 12kg.

The dose of adrenaline (epinephrine) is 0.1mL/kg of 1 in10 000 (10μg/kg of body weight).

Appendix 7 shows the UK Resuscitation Council's paediatric advanced life support algorithm.

→ http://www.resus.org.uk/pages/pals.pdf

41. B ★ ★ ★ ★   OHEM, 4th edn → p734

According to the formula described above, the boy's approximate body weight is 24kg.

In trauma cases, crystalloid is given at the rate of 10mL/kg body weight in boluses. Therefore, the initial bolus of fluid should be 240mL. It may be repeated if necessary. Consider giving blood if the child requires more than 40mL/kg of fluid.

42. C ★ ★ ★ ★   OHEM, 4th edn → p736

Because the spine in children is elastic, spinal cord injuries may occur without radiographic abnormalities (SCIWORA). The history of neck pain following an injury with numbness, pins and needles or focal sign should not be ignored even if the cervical spine X-ray is normal. A normal cervical spine series may be found in up to two-thirds of children who have experienced a spinal cord injury.

A: Cervical cord injury is relatively less common in children in comparison with adults. Cervical spine immobilization is required if a child is involved in road traffic collisions or sporting activities.

B: See above.

D: Ligaments are elastic in children, therefore, such injuries are uncommon.

E: The onset of objective signs of the cord injury may be delayed, therefore, any transient neurological symptoms must be taken seriously.

American College of Surgeons Committee on Trauma (2008) *Advanced Trauma Life Support for Doctors, Student Course Manual*, 8th edn. American College of Surgeons, p241.

43. D ★ ★ ★   OHEM, 4th edn → p746

Between the age of 1 and 5 years, a direct pull on the long axis of the forearm distally may cause the subluxation of the radial head (radial head out of the annular ligament). It is more common in girls than boys and the left elbow more than the right one. The child is reluctant to move the arm, which is held in slight flexion at the elbow and the child is unable to supinate the forearm. In the presence of a typical history, there is no need for X-ray. The subluxation can be reduced easily by exertion of light pressure on the radial head by the examiner's thumb and supinating the forearm and flexing the elbow in one motion, maintaining slight traction by holding the hand. A click is often felt when the radial head is reduced.

A: Dislocation of the elbow occurs when the patient falls on an outstretched hand with elbow extended at the time of the fall.

B: Olecranon fracture is less common in children than adults. The mechanism of such an injury is either direct impact as a result of a fall or road traffic collision.

C: The mechanism of this injury is fall on an outstretched hand.

E: This occurs following a fall on the outstretched hand with the hyperextended elbow causing the distal fragment of the humerus to displace in the proximal and posterior direction resulting in an extension type of supracondylar fracture. The flexion type of fracture occurs following a direct blow to the flexed elbow.

44. C ★ ★ ★   OHEM, 4th edn → p232

The child is clinically shocked with a reduced level of consciousness, pale skin, cold extremities, tachycardia, tachypnoea and prolonged capillary refill. The child should be given 0.9% normal saline or 0.9% normal saline with 5% dextrose 20mL/kg body weight and the response monitored. Both fluid deficit replacement and maintenance may be treated using the same type of crystalloid. Maintenance fluids should be given according to the body weight (for the first 10kg body weight use 100mL/kg, second 10kg 50mL/kg and subsequent kg 20mL/kg). So the maintenance fluid requirement for this child is 1000 + 100 = 1100mL/24h.

A: Measure the urea, creatinine, sodium, potassium, and glucose at the outset and alter the fluid composition or rate of administration if necessary, but the initial therapy should not wait for the blood results.

B: The NICE guideline (see weblink below) suggests that a crystalloid (as mentioned below) should be started.

D: The child has decreased level of consciousness and repeated vomiting, and so would not tolerate the oral rehydration therapy.

E: The child is dehydrated and requires IV fluids urgently. Stool microscopy is not helpful in this situation. The indications for sending stool culture are:

- Suspected septicaemia
- Blood and/or mucus in the stool
- The child is immunocompromised.

→ www.nice.org.uk/nicemedia/pdf/CG84FullGuideline.pdf (see p20, Flow chart of fluid management).

45. C ★ ★ ★ ★ OHEM, 4th edn → pp664–5

The baby has not responded to initial five breaths. The positions of the head should be checked (neutral position) and then jaw thrust tried followed by five inflation breaths. Confirm response by visible chest movements or increase in heart rate.

A: Adrenaline (epinephrine) should only be given after the chest compression is started (as a part of advanced life support protocol).

B: As hypoxia is the commonest cause of bradycardia in children (including infants and newborns), atropine must not be given.

D: Cardiac compression is started if the heart rate drops below 60bpm.

E: Suction should be performed if the baby has not responded to C and a second person called to maintain the airway.

Immediately after birth, wrap (without drying) and place the baby under radiant heat. Set a clock in motion and assess colour, tone, breathing and pulse (Apgar score, see Table 15.5).

For additional information, see the *Oxford Handbook of Clinical Specialties*, 8th edn, p107 and the *Oxford Handbook of Paediatrics*, p114.

Fig. 15.14 shows a flow chart of neonatal resuscitation (source: The UK Resuscitation Guidelines 2010, the newborn life support, page 121 of NLS – the web page is http://www.resus.org.uk/pages/nls.pdf). For a large version of this figure, please visit the book's Online Resource Centre.

Wrap (without drying) and place under radiant heat

↓

Initial assesment; set a clock in motion; assess *colour, tone, breathing, and pluse*. If not breathing after ~90s

↓

Control the airway (head in the neutral position)

↓

Support breathing: 5 inflation breaths; 3s long. Confirm response: visible chest movements or ↑heart rate

↓

If no response, check *head position* and try a *jaw thrust*; then 5 inflation breaths.
Confirm response: visible chest movement or ↑heart rate

↓

If still no response, get 2nd person to help with airway control and inflation breaths.
Any sucking out of the pharynx should be better direct vision

- Repeat 5 inflation breaths
- Insert oropharyngeal airway
- Repeat inflation breaths

Consider intubation. Confirm response: visible chest movement or increased heart rate

↓

When chest is moving, continue with ventilation breaths if no spontaneous breathing.

↓

Check heart rate; if absent or <60 (and not rising) *start chest compressions*. Do 3 chest
compressions to 1 breath, for 30s

↓

Reasess pulse: if improving stop chest compression. If not breathing, go on ventilating. If heart rate still↓
continue ventilation and chest compressions

↓

Consider IV or umbilical access and drugs, e.g. adrenaline (epinephrine): 100µg/kg (0.1mL 1:10 000/kg)IV.

▶At all stages ask *Do I need help?*

Table 15.5 The Apgar score

Apgar	Pulse	Respirations	Muscle tone	Colour	On suction
2	>100	Strong cry	Active	Pink	Coughs well
1	<100	Slow, irregular	Limb flexion	Blue limbs	Depressed cough
0	0	Nil	Absent	All blue or white	No response

Source: *Oxford Handbook of Clinical Specialties.*

46. E ★★★★ OHEM, 4th edn → pp701–3

With minimal improvement as in the case above, it is advisable to repeat the nebulized salbutamol along with nebulized ipratropium bromide 0.25mg. Salbutamol is an adrenergic drug, which leads to bronchodilation through stimulation of β_2 receptors, whereas ipratropium bromide is anticholinergic drug and blocks reflex bronchoconstriction and reverses acute airway obstruction. Its onset of action is slower than β_2 agonists, so ipratropium bromide should not be used alone in acute asthma.

A: Although the child has not improved much, he has not deteriorated either; call for paediatrician or paediatric intensive care team only if he develops life-threatening features.

B: Such cases with severe asthma are not safe to discharge and may require hospitalization under a paediatrician as they often require continuous treatment and monitoring.

C: Antibiotics should not be given 'routinely' if there is no specific indication of sepsis or infection. A bolus of IV salbutamol may be given if the child develops life-threatening features.

D: IV aminophylline is not recommended in children with mild to moderate asthma. Aminophylline may be considered after taking specialist advice only in the cases of severe or life-threatening asthma unresponsive to maximal doses of bronchodilators and systemic steroids.

Fig. 15.15 shows the normal peak expiratory flow rates in children aged 5–18 years.

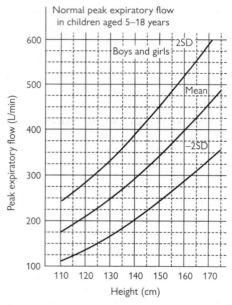

→ www.brit-thoracic.org.uk

→ www.sign.ac.uk/pdf/sign101.pdf (**Go to Annex 6**)

47. E ★ ★ ★ ★ OHEM, 4th edn → p698

Westley croup score is calculated by adding the following individual values:

1. Stridor:

   a. None = 0

   b. Only when upset or agitated = 1

at rest = 2

oxygen saturation <92% on air/cyanosis:

  a. None = 0

  b. With agitation = 4

  c. At rest = 5

3. Level of consciousness:

  a. Normal = 0

  b. Altered mental state = 5

4. Air entry:

  a. Normal = 0

  b. Decreased = 1

  c. Markedly decreased = 2

5. Retraction:

  a. None = 0

  b. Mild = 1

  c. At rest = 2

The maximum score is 16.

Mild croup (0–1) = many of these children can be discharged.

Moderate (2–7) = may require hospital admission; give an oral dose of dexamethasone or budesonide nebulized, both of which can be used in mild cases as well.

Severe (>7) = the child may need nebulized adrenaline (epinephrine), driven by oxygen, and will require admission.

Westley CR, Cotton EK, Brooks JG (1978) Nebulized racemic adrenaline by IPPB for the treatment of croup: a double-blind study. *Am J Dis Child* **132**(5):484–7.

→ http://clinicalevidence.bmj.com/ceweb/conditions/chd/0321/0321_background.jsp

48. A ★ ★ ★ ★ OHEM, 4th edn → pp741, 749

This is a type III injury according to the Salter–Harris classification of epiphyseal injury. It carries a moderate risk of long term complications. As it is undisplaced, the ankle should be immobilized in a back slab, a check X-ray performed to ensure no displacement has occurred and the patient referred to the next fracture clinic. Such fractures when displaced require immediate referral to the on-call orthopaedics team for accurate open reduction and internal fixation.

For the reason mentioned above, the other options are inappr...
The risks of long-term growth problems are lower in types I and...
undisplaced injuries than types III–V injuries.

49. A ★ ★ ★ ★ OHEM, 4th edn → pp490, 749

This patient has a patellar dislocation. Following a direct blow on the medial side, the patella typically dislocates laterally. The painful knee is held in slight flexion and the patella visibly dislocated laterally. The patient complaints of inability to flex the knee. It should be reduced immediately using Entonox inhalation. IV analgesia is not generally required. Request X-rays after reduction and then immobilize in a cylinder cast. Check the X-ray carefully for a small osteochondral chip fracture of the undersurface of the patella.
The patient should be followed up in the next fracture clinic. Immediate reduction is also associated with relief of pain. A junior doctor while seeing such case for the first time, may require help from an experienced ED doctor.

B: The patient does not require referral to the orthopaedics on-call team.

C and D: Simple Tubigrip application or back slab immobilization is not advocated as reduction as early as possible is of paramount importance.

E: X-ray before reduction is not recommended as the diagnosis is usually obvious and reduction should not be delayed. The longer the joint is left unreduced, the more damage is done. It also relieves the pain almost immediately.

Extended Matching Answers

1. D ★ OHEM, 4th edn → p686

The patient has Henoch–Schönlein purpura, in which the vasculitic process affects small arteries in the kidneys, skin, and GI tract. It is relatively common in 4–11 year olds and appears to follow a viral or bacterial infection. Erythematous macules develop into palpable purpuric lesions, which are characteristically concentrated over the buttocks and extensor surfaces of the lower limbs. Joint pains in the knees and ankles with abdominal pain may be associated features. Nephritis may occur producing microscopic and macroscopic haematuria and proteinuria.

2. E ★ ★ OHEM, 4th edn → p686

About 4 in every 100 000 children develop idiopathic thrombocytopenic purpura each year. There seem to be two groups who develop this disease: young children (2–4 years) and young adults. It is also three times more common in girls than boys. The actual cause is unknown but probably follows a viral infection as a result of an autoimmune reaction. The patient presents with a purpuric rash, mucous membrane bleeding, conjunctival haemorrhages and sometimes GI bleeding. The platelet count is usually <30×10⁹/L.

→ www.ich.ucl.ac.uk/gosh_families/information_sheets/idiopathic_ thrombocytopenic_purpura/idiopathic_thrombocytopenic_purpura_ families.html

3. A ★ ★   OHEM, 4th edn → p686

Acute lymphoblastic leukaemia accounts for 80% of leukaemias in children. In most children, leukaemia presents insidiously over several weeks, but in some, it may progress rapidly. The blood count is abnormal in most cases with a low haemoglobin, thrombocytopenia, and circulating blast cells. Bone marrow examination is essential to confirm the diagnosis.

Lissauer T, Clayden G (2001) *Illustrated Textbook of Paediatrics*, 2nd edn. Edinburgh: Mosby.

4. I ★   OHEM, 4th edn → p686

The purpura has developed as a result of coughing and retching, diagnosed by its localized distribution in the face area, caused by increased pressure in the tributaries of superior vena cava. Back pressure causes the petechiae to develop. The blood results are normal in such cases.

5. H ★   OHEM, 4th edn → pp688–91

The patient has meningococcal septicaemia. She is unwell with purpuric rashes. Meningococcal disease may present as septicaemia, meningitis, or rash. The disease may be well advanced if it presents with rash. This may be initially blanching, macular, or maculopapular. The petechial or purpuric rash may be a very late sign and carry a very poor prognosis.

→ www.meningitis.org

6. A ★   OHEM, 4th edn → p721

These features are typical of acute appendicitis. Such patients should be referred to the surgeons for further management.

Lissauer T, Clayden G (2001) *Illustrated Textbook of Paediatrics* 2nd edn. Edinburgh: Mosby.

Williams NS, Bulstrode CJK, O'Connell PR (eds) (2008). *Bailey & Love's Short Practice of Surgery*, 25th edn. London: Hodder Arnold.

7. B ★★   OHEM, 4th edn → p522

The clinical features are similar to acute appendicitis but the pain is poorly localized, not aggravated by movements, and rarely accompanied by guarding. The site of severity of maximum tenderness often varies during the course of repeated examinations. Symptoms are typically self-limiting within 48h. The aetiology of non-specific abdominal pain in children is obscure but viral infections may account for some cases. Such patients may be admitted under a paediatrician for observation. The diagnosis of mesenteric adenitis can only be made definitively in those children in whom large mesenteric nodes are seen at laparotomy or laparoscopy and whose appendix is normal.

Lissauer T, Clayden G (2001) *Illustrated Textbook of Paediatrics*, 2nd edn. Edinburgh: Mosby.

Williams NS, Bulstrode CJK, O'Connell PR (eds) (2008). *Bailey & Love's Short Practice of Surgery*, 25th edn. London: Hodder Arnold.

8. E ★★   OHEM, 4th edn → p720

There is hypertrophy of the circular muscle layer of the pylorus after being born with normal pylorus. Boys are affected four times more than girls. It typically presents between 2 and 7 weeks. Patients presents with non-bilious projectile vomiting. Ultrasound examination may confirm the diagnosis. A hypochloraemic alkalosis with low serum potassium may be present because of vomiting of the stomach contents and this must be corrected before surgery.

Lissauer T, Clayden G (2001) *Illustrated Textbook of Paediatrics*, 2nd edn. Edinburgh: Mosby.

Williams NS, Bulstrode CJK, O'Connell PR (eds) (2008). *Bailey & Love's Short Practice of Surgery*, 25th edn. London: Hodder Arnold.

9. G ★★   OHEM, 4th edn → p721

Intussusception occurs at any age and in both sexes with a peak incidence between 5 and 12 months. The classical triad is pain, vomiting, and per rectal bleeding. Only one third of the patients will have all the three features and three-quarters will have two of these symptoms. Intussusception should be considered in any infant with a bloody stool. A sausage-shaped mass is often palpable in the abdomen. Intussusception is the commonest cause of intestinal obstruction in infants after the neonatal period. Diagnosis may be confirmed by ultrasound scan or contrast enema. Shock is an important complication of intussusception. In infantile hypertrophic pyloric stenosis, the vomitus does not have bile.

Lissauer T, Clayden G (2001) *Illustrated Textbook of Paediatrics*, 2nd edn. Edinburgh: Mosby.

Williams NS, Bulstrode CJK, O'Connell PR (eds) (2008). *Bailey & Love's Short Practice of Surgery*, 25th edn. London: Hodder Arnold.

10. D ★ OHEM, 4th edn → p230

The most likely diagnosis is gastroenteritis. If in doubt the patient may be admitted for observation and given oral rehydration therapy. The most common cause is rotavirus.

Lissauer T, Clayden G (2001) *Illustrated Textbook of Paediatrics*, 2nd edn. Edinburgh: Mosby.

Williams NS, Bulstrode CJK, O'Connell PR (eds) (2008). *Bailey & Love's Short Practice of Surgery*, 25th edn. London: Hodder Arnold.

11. B ★★

Most of the antibiotics cause low-grade toxicity. Such patients may be allowed home after initial assessment and discussion with parents about keeping the medication safe at home. Large doses may cause nausea, vomiting, and skin rashes. Hypersensitivity reactions may occur. Large IV dose of penicillin may cause convulsions.

Lissauer T, Clayden G (2001) *Illustrated Textbook of Paediatrics*, 2nd edn. Edinburgh: Mosby.

→ www.toxbase.org/Poisons-Index-A-Z/A-Products/Amoxicillin/

12. G ★★

Household bleach is a mild to moderate irritant, which does not cause tissue damage unless ingested in large amounts. Ingestion of more than 100mL in a child or 300mL in an adult of household bleach may cause significant toxicity. Most patients will have no more than minimal features of toxicity, unless a large amount has been ingested (haematemesis, retrosternal chest pain because of corrosive oesophagitis, etc.). Small amounts cause a burning sensation in the mouth and throat, and thirst. The oropharynx may be mildly inflamed but burns are unlikely. Nausea, retching, vomiting, diarrhoea, and haematemesis may occur but are unlikely to be severe. Occasionally there may be signs of pulmonary irritant effects such as cough, wheeze, or dyspnoea. So, after observing the child for a couple of hours he may be discharged if the above features are absent, once he has had his feeds and has been able to keep them down.

→ www.toxbase.org/Poisons-Index-A-Z/H-Products/Sodium-Hypochlorite-Solution/

13. F ★★

Usually no treatment is required, but aspiration pneumonitis may develop. Emesis in contraindicated. Monitor on the paediatric ward.

→ www.toxbase.org/Poisons-Index-A-Z/W-Products/White-Spirit/

14. A ★★   OHEM, 4th edn → pp718–9, 193

Within an hour of ingestion of paracetamol, she should be given activated charcoal 25g. The blood paracetamol level should be measured at 4h after the ingestion and treatment with antidote (*N*-acetylcysteine) should be started if required (guided by the blood levels).

→ www.toxbase.org/Poisons-Index-A-Z/P-Products/
Paracetamol------------/

15. F ★★   OHEM, 4th edn → p404

The patient's GCS score is 12/15 (E3, V4, and M5) because of the alcohol overdose. The bedside capillary blood glucose test should be done to rule out hypoglycaemia and normal saline infusion started. She must be observed on a ward and her blood alcohol level may be measured for checking severity. Once she has recovered a detailed history should be taken to confirm that this was only a one-off episode and there is no underlying problem of recurrent alcohol abuse.

→ www.toxbase.org/Poisons-Index-A-Z/A-Products/Alcohol/

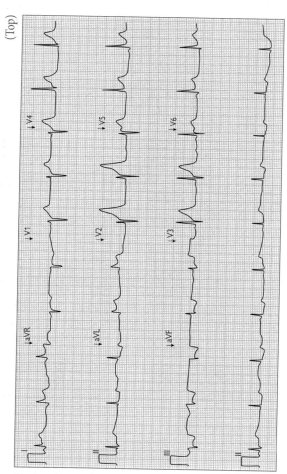

Fig. 3.1 (see p 39).

(Top)

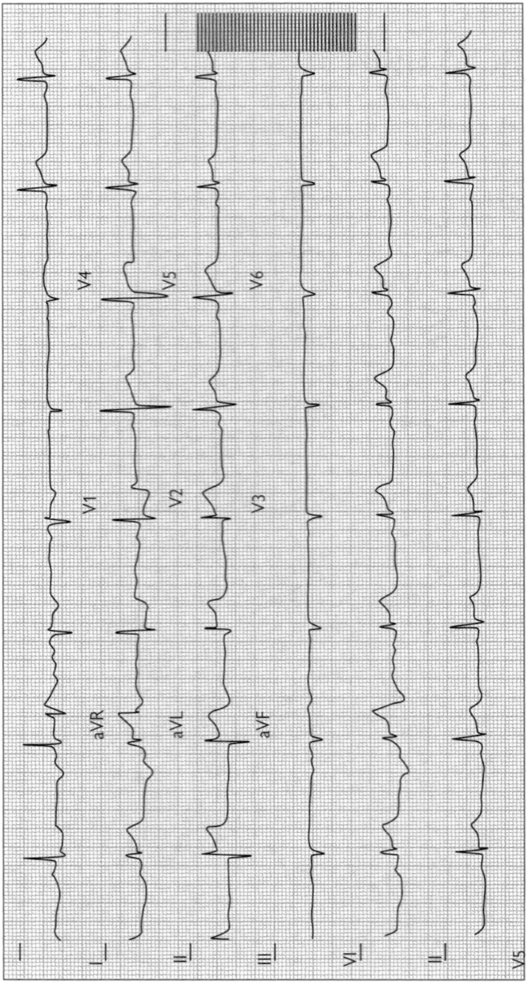

Fig. 3.2 (see p 40).

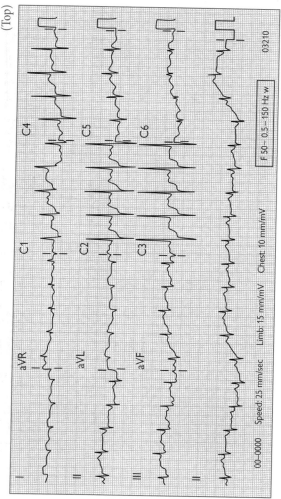

Fig. 3.3 (see p 41).

(Top)

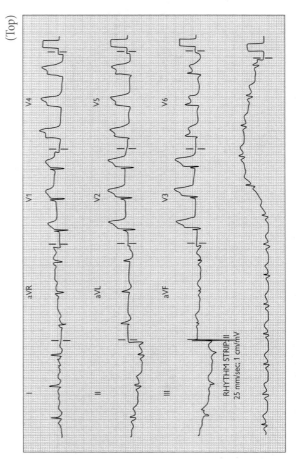

Fig. 3.4 (see p 42).

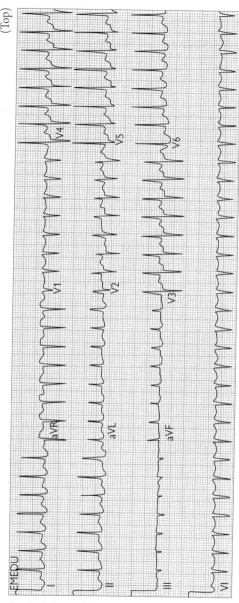

(Top)

Fig. 3.11 (see p 68).

403

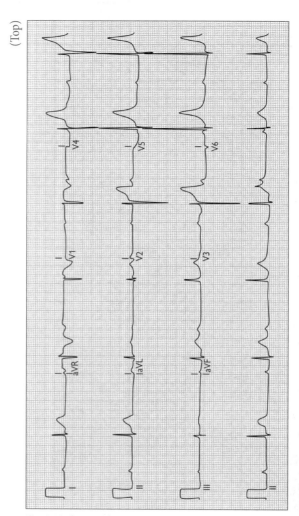

Fig. 3.12 (see p 68).

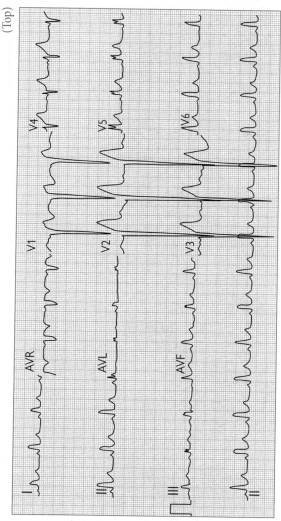

(Top)

Fig. 3.21 (see p 96).

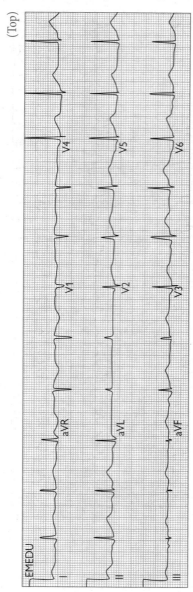

(Top)

Fig. 3.22 (see p 96).

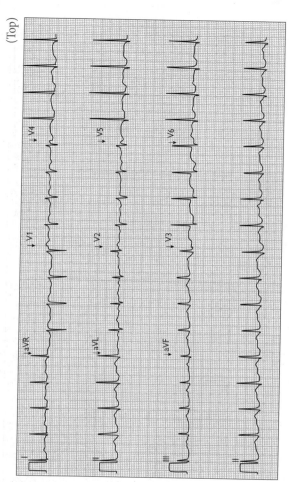

Fig. 3.23 (see p 97).

(Top)

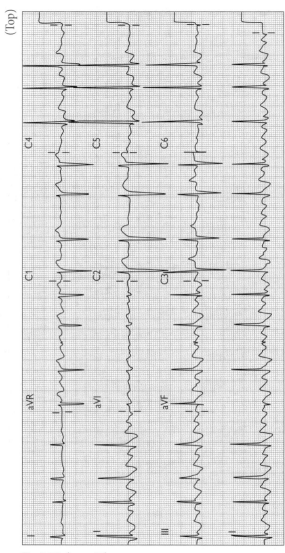

Fig. 3.24 (see p 97).

408

APPENDIX 1
ANAPHYLAXIS ALGORITHM, JANUARY 2008

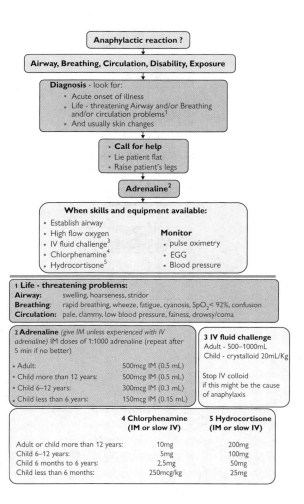

Anaphylactic reaction ?

Airway, Breathing, Circulation, Disability, Exposure

Diagnosis - look for:
- Acute onset of illness
- Life - threatening Airway and/or Breathing and/or circulation problems[1]
- And usually skin changes

- **Call for help**
- Lie patient flat
- Raise patient's legs

Adrenaline[2]

When skills and equipment available:
- Establish airway
- High flow oxygen
- IV fluid challenge[3]   **Monitor**
- Chlorphenamine[4]   - pulse oximetry
- Hydrocortisone[5]   - EGG
                                - Blood pressure

1 Life - threatening problems:
Airway: swelling, hoarseness, stridor
Breathing: rapid breathing, wheeze, fatigue, cyanosis, SpO$_2$< 92%, confusion
Circulation: pale, clammy, low blood pressure, fainess, drowsy/coma

2 Adrenaline *(give IM unless experienced with IV adrenaline)* IM doses of 1:1000 adrenaline (repeat after 5 min if no better)

• Adult:	500mcg IM (0.5 mL)
• Child more than 12 years:	500mcg IM (0.5 mL)
• Child 6–12 years:	300mcg IM (0.3 mL)
• Child less than 6 years:	150mcg IM (0.15 mL)

3 IV fluid challenge
Adult - 500–1000mL
Child - crystalloid 20mL/Kg

Stop IV colloid
if this might be the cause
of anaphylaxis

	4 Chlorphenamine (IM or slow IV)	5 Hydrocortisone (IM or slow IV)
Adult or child more than 12 years:	10mg	200mg
Child 6–12 years:	5mg	100mg
Child 6 months to 6 years:	2.5mg	50mg
Child less than 6 months:	250mcg/kg	25mg

ADULT BASIC LIFE SUPPORT ALGORITHM, OCTOBER 2010

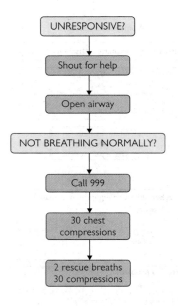

UNRESPONSIVE?

Shout for help

Open airway

NOT BREATHING NORMALLY?

Call 999

30 chest compressions

2 rescue breaths 30 compressions

APPENDIX 3
ALS ALGORITHM, OCTOBER 2010

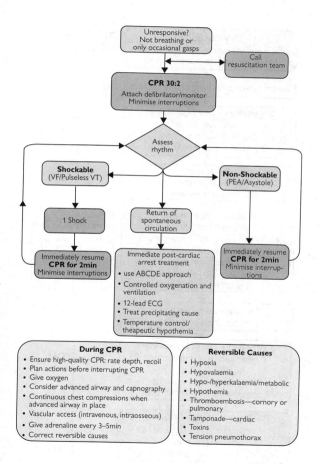

APPENDIX 4
NEWBORN LIFE SUPPORT, OCTOBER 2010

Dry the baby Remove any wet towels and cover Start the clock or note the time	Birth	AT
Assess (tone), breathing and heart rate	30 s	ALL
If gasping or **not breathing:** Open the airway Give 5 inflation breaths consider SpO$_2$ monitoring	60 s	STAGES
Re-assess if no increase in heart rate look for chest movement		ASK:

If chest not moving: Recheck head position Consider 2-person airway control and other airway manoeuvres Repeat inflation breaths Consider SpO$_2$ monitoring Look for a response	Acceptable* pre-ductal SpO$_2$ 2min 60% 3min 70% 4min 80% 5min 85% 10min 90%

If no increase in heart rate look for chest movement	DO
When the chest is moving: If heart rate is not detectable or slow (<60min^{-1}) Start chest compressions 3 compressions to each breath	YOU
	NEED
Reassess heart rate every 30s if heart rate is not detectable or slow (<60min^{-1}) consider venous access and drugs	HELP?

* See Dawson JA, Kamlin CO, Vento M, et al. Defining the reference range for oxygen saturation for infants after birth. *Pediatrics* 2010;125:e1340–7.

PAEDIATRIC BASIC LIFE SUPPORT, OCTOBER 2010

(Healthcare professionals with a duty to respond)

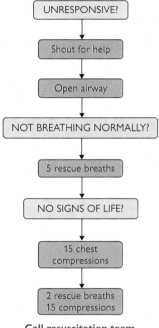

Call resuscitation team

APPENDIX 6
PAEDIATRIC CHOKING TREATMENT ALGORITHM, OCTOBER 2010

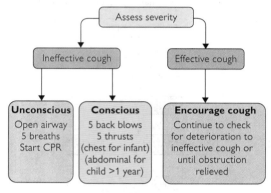

Safety and summoning assistance

Safety is paramount. Rescuers should avoid placing themselves in danger and consider the safest action to manage the choking child:

- If the child is coughing effectively, then no external manoeuvre is necessary. Encourage the child to cough, and monitor continuously.
- If the child's coughing is, or is becoming, ineffective, **shout for help** immediately and determine the child's conscious level.

PAEDIATRIC ADVANCED LIFE SUPPORT, OCTOBER 2010

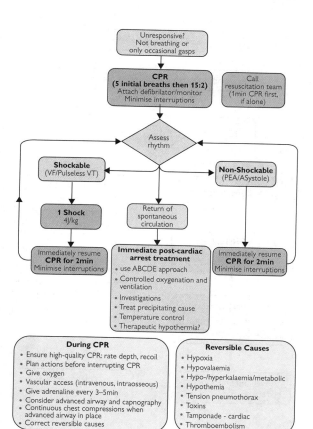

Unresponsive?
Not breathing or
only occasional gasps

CPR
(5 initial breaths then 15:2)
Attach defibrilator/monitor
Minimise interruptions

Call
resuscitation team
(1min CPR first,
if alone)

Assess rhythm

Shockable
(VF/Pulseless VT)

Non-Shockable
(PEA/ASystole)

1 Shock
4J/kg

Return of
spontaneous
circulation

Immediately resume
CPR for 2min
Minimise interruptions

Immediate post-cardiac
arrest treatment
• use ABCDE approach
• Controlled oxygenation and
ventilation
• Investigations
• Treat precipitating cause
• Temperature control
• Therapeutic hypothermia?

Immediately resume
CPR for 2min
Minimise interruptions

During CPR
• Ensure high-quality CPR: rate depth, recoil
• Plan actions before interrupting CPR
• Give oxygen
• Vascular access (intravenous, intraosseous)
• Give adrenaline every 3–5min
• Consider advanced airway and capnography
• Continuous chest compressions when
advanced airway in place
• Correct reversible causes

Reversible Causes
• Hypoxia
• Hypovalaemia
• Hypo-/hyperkalaemia/metabolic
• Hypothemia
• Tension pneumothorax
• Toxins
• Tamponade - cardiac
• Thromboembolism

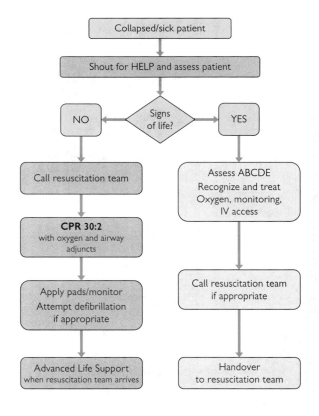

Collapsed/sick patient

Shout for HELP and assess patient

NO — Signs of life? — YES

NO branch:

Call resuscitation team

CPR 30:2
with oxygen and airway adjuncts

Apply pads/monitor
Attempt defibrillation if appropriate

Advanced Life Support
when resuscitation team arrives

YES branch:

Assess ABCDE
Recognize and treat
Oxygen, monitoring,
IV access

Call resuscitation team
if appropriate

Handover
to resuscitation team

GLASGOW COMA SCALE (ADULTS)

Eye response	open spontaneously	4
	open to verbal command	3
	open to pain	2
	no response	1
Verbal response	talking and orientated	5
	confused/disorientated	4
	inappropriate words	3
	incomprehensible sounds	2
	no response	1
Motor response	obeys commands	6
	localizes pain	5
	flexion/withdrawal	4
	abnormal flexion	3
	extension	2
	no response	1
Total (GCS)	Range 3–15	

INDEX